FIRST TIME MOM'S SURVIVAL HANDBOOK

How to Prepare Yourself for Healthy Pregnancy, Labor, Childbirth, Newborn and Motherhood

Deja-Brook Ransome

Ransome Unlimited

CONTENTS

INTRODUCTION

Hello future Mommy,

I would like to welcome you on this lifelong journey of motherhood. I know at times it can seem daunting, and maybe a little scary, but I am here to happily hold your hand when you have feelings of uncertainty. I want you to be excited about this journey and that is only possible through being well-informed. I want you to move away from survival mode to thriving throughout your pregnancy and your lifelong journey. The word pregnancy originates from the Latin words praegnant simply meaning before birth (Merriam-Webster, 2020). The word pregnancy is associated with many things such as growing bellies, swollen feet and food cravings. Your pregnancy journey will be similar to that of many, but every journey is unique and deeply personal. I want you to view this guide as a helpful friend who wants nothing more than to see you happy and fulfilled. On average 350,000 babies are born a day to what I imagine to be slightly scared, a little anxious and very expectant parents. That's an average of 243 babies per minute. So while you are watching an episode of your favorite show or preparing dinner, someone else's life is changing. This illustrates the difference a minute can make in someone's life.

Women experience pressure from all angles of their lives especially when it comes to when they are expected to have children. This pressure to procreate often comes from those closest to us, like our friends and family. They will justify their opinions by saying that they just want what's best for you, or that you need to take your internal clock more seriously. This constant reminder of a woman's internal clock often feels like a dark cloud hovering over all of our heads. They might have good intentions, but I need you to understand that **no one** can make this decision for you. If you get to the end of this book and decide that children are not in your plans anymore, that's okay and completely your choice. Motherhood is not a phase that you should rush into or take lightly. I understand that at times it feels like everywhere you look, you see adorable newborn babies. Mommy influencers and old friends will have you convinced that they are the perfect parents through their posts. You'll see pictures on social media of perfectly round bellies, regal pregnancy shoots and perfectly tiny hands and feet. I need you to ignore the social media pressure and understand that every journey is different, so silence all the pressures and mentally reset your internal clock. I know that pregnancy can seem scary, and trust me your fears are all valid and understandable. It can be hard and understandably a little overwhelming to fully wrap your head around the idea of a person growing inside of you.

If you take a moment to put all your fears and anxious

feelings aside, then you can see pregnancy for what it is, an exciting new chapter. A chapter that I cannot wait for you to experience. New parents and family members all anxiously waiting to find out if you are having a boy or girl. Everyone will be rushing to see who the baby looks like and if all ten fingers and toes are accounted for. The nights you'll spend wondering about your child's personality and whether they'll take your good or bad traits. Pregnancy is a euphoric experience that is often difficult to fully put into words. It is transformative and understandably life-altering. I may not know what your beliefs are, but I believe that pregnancy is a universal unifier because it is present in everyone's journey toward motherhood regardless of if they carry the child themselves. It is a beautiful process that allows you to transition into a new phase of your life. You are on a journey that will at times feel overwhelming, but trust me it's worth the memories and the milestones you will help foster and capture. Think of it this way: you are litterally ensuring the continuation of human existence. Amazing!

This book is titled *First Time Mom's Survival Handbook* for a reason, so expect to find all the information that you need to know within these pages. This book will take you through every step on your pregnancy journey. The goal of this guide is to leave you feeling informed and ready to take on this journey without any hesitation. I want you to feel confident in your abilities and develop skills that will assist you throughout your journey. I'm with you from the moment you decide that motherhood is right for you. I will offer advice and some wisdom on how to properly prepare yourself and those around you for this new phase. It will enable you to effectively plan for your future by providing clear steps on the methods you can take to reach your destination. I will discuss everything from how to prepare your mind, body and spirit to ensure a healthy pregnancy. We will look at the main themes often associated with pregnancy such as what you can expect from labor, childbirth, handling a newborn and motherhood. I want you to get comfortable with these themes so that when the time comes you are ready and comfortable.

We will talk about everything from when the right time to see your doctor is, cracked nipples, stretch marks, all the way to deciding on baby names. The key is to take everything step by step and not rush into anything. Congratulations on joining an ever-growing group of modern mothers who want to effectively manage their pregnancy journey. Welcome to the mom tribe! I'm happy to take this journey with you.

CHAPTER 1: PREPARATION TIME:

Get Yourself Together

It all starts with making the crucial decision that motherhood is for you. Once you have made that decision, it's time to prepare. I am sure you have heard the popular phrase that in order to be successful, preparation is key. This statement is especially crucial when it comes to pregnancy. It all starts with getting yourself together, because as I am sure you already know you are a crucial component to pregnancy. Let's start with preparing your body through physical exercise and diet.

It's important to understand the role that your body will play throughout your pregnancy. It's helpful to imagine pregnancy as a visit from a dear friend. Your friend tells you that they are going to be visiting you in a few months and asks if it's okay for them to stay in your home. You are understandably excited and since this is one of your very good friends you spend months preparing for the visit to ensure that they have a pleasant stay. You make sure that the guest room is tidy and that the bed is perfectly made. You consider their dietary requirements and plan activities that you know they will enjoy. You do all of this because you want to be a good host and you care about your friend. Your womb will provide a home for your child throughout your pregnancy, so you want to do everything you possibly can to make sure that it is a pleasant stay for your child. You make sure that you're a good host to your unborn child the same way you would prepare for an old friend. Physical exercise allows you to prepare yourself for the journey.

Physical exercise simply means living an active life that leads to a healthier lifestyle. It has been found that physical exercise has a positive impact on a woman's fertility. You are more likely to have fewer issues with regards to your fertility when your body mass index is at a normal level. It allows you to have a higher chance of falling pregnant without any medical assistance. Your body mass index refers to a rating scale that takes into consideration your weight and height. It determines whether your weight is at a normal level or if you are obese (Westaway, 2016). The physical exercise you partake in is not to promote weight loss but for general healthier levels of activity.

A program called Your Fertility by the Australian government to promote healthy lifestyles during pregnancy found that exercise plays a key role in conception (Fertility, 2012). It is advised that women exercise for a minimum of 30 minutes a day to promote a healthier lifestyle. I know that 30 minutes can seem daunting but exercise can take many different forms. You can take a walk through your neighbourhood, have a solo dance party to some of your favourite tunes or follow an at-home workout plan. The idea of working out does not need to be boring, so try making it fun for yourself. You can do this by asking your friends to try a new dance class with you or by going out and buying yourself new workout gear. It's important to get your mindset right before exercising and wearing the correct attire can help shift your mindset. The key is to not overly exert yourself but practice moderate amounts of exercise. I'm sure it's a relief to hear that you don't have to train like an Olympian or professional athlete, because that can cause more harm than good. You can tell if you are overdoing your exercise routine by being aware of your body. If you feel overly exhausted and often light-headed, chances are, you are straining yourself. A key sign that you are overworking yourself is joint pain. If you keep a lookout for these signs you are sure to not overwork yourself(de Bellefonds, 2018). The key is to find your balance for you to have normal activity levels. The reason you are including daily exercise in your daily routine before conception is because you want to create healthy habits that you can continue throughout your pregnancy. It's also vital that your partner partakes in moderate levels of exercise as it improves the quality of the sperm he produces; both of you must be physically healthy (Fertility, 2012). The quality of his sperm directly impacts your chances of conception as well as your child's well-being.

The next factor that you need to take into consideration is altering your diet. You need to incorporate healthy eating habits into your routine. This will allow you to continue these habits throughout your pregnancy and after you give birth. It is important to have a sufficient intake of vitamins and nutrients throughout your journey. Be intentional about avoiding caffeine, alcohol and cigarettes during this time, as it negatively affects your health. Studies now show that pregnant women can safely consume 200mg of caffeine per day. This amounts to two cups of coffee a day and if you're still apprehensive about drinking coffee try switching to a decaffeinated version. Simply because you no longer drink alcohol that doesn't mean that you need to cut out girls nights. There are several non-alcoholic drink options at bars that you can enjoy while out with your friends. Your friends will be glad to hear that for the next few months they don't have to take turns being the designated driver. This service might win you a few free babysitting sessions from your friends later on. It is important to make these changes because it allows you to find more positive ways to regain your energy. You have to remain conscious of the fact that your health directly affects that of your child even before conception. A study by Kids Health (2016) found that your health prior to conception is vital. You should aim to eat a balanced diet that includes a variety of food. Your diet should include a sufficient amount of fruits, vegetables, starch and protein. Similar to incorporating exercise into your schedule, a healthy diet should also be incorporated gradually. Look at your current eating habits and decide what you can effortlessly do away with. It might seem less daunting to alter your entire eating structure if you start with a few items at a time. I suggest doing away with unnecessary snacks initially. Instead of binging on sweets, chocolates and chips try healthier alternatives such as vegetable chips or fruit. The aim is to simply consume unhealthy items less frequently. If eating healthy snacks becomes a habit in your daily life, then it's easier to carry this behavior into your other meals. It's important to remember that eating healthy meals does not mean that your meals have to be boring. This change allows you the opportunity to try out new recipes and be more creative in the kitchen. Consider this an exciting new journey that you can include your partner in; both of you need to make changes to your diet in order to increase your chances of conceiving a healthy child. It is important to consume enough healthy liquids throughout this journey as well. It is advised that you drink at least 6 cups of water a day because it helps your organs function and removes toxins from your body (Sick Kids Staff, 2016).

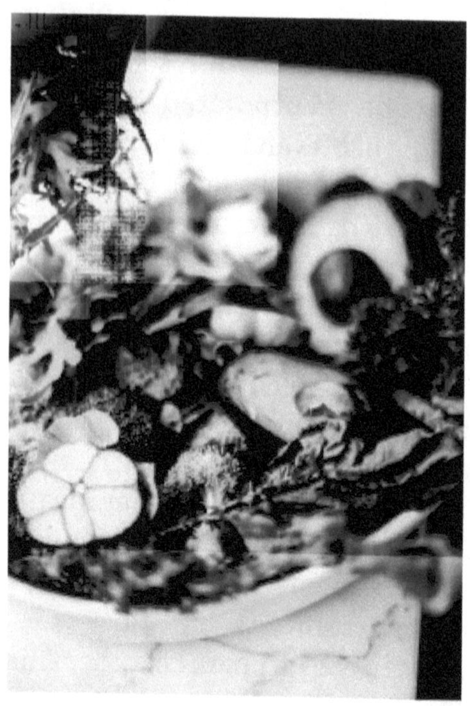

Mommies, I know that these might seem like difficult changes, but I will suggest easy foods that you should incorporate into your diet. To improve your chances of conception, there are a few staples you can add to your diet. A good rule of thumb to live by is including more green vegetables into your diet. The greener the better, so go for vegetables like spinach, kale or broccoli. You can consume these vegetables in a variety of ways, like in your breakfast as an ingredient in your omelette or as a side salad for your dinner or lunch. Seasonal fruits are a great source of vitamins. Citrus fruits are a great addition to your diet, such as oranges or grapefruit.

Citrus has been found to assist in combating morning sickness. It is important that you consume all of these foods in moderation, especially dairy products. Dairy is beneficial prior to conception because it allows your reproductive system to function correctly. Your calcium levels are vital throughout your pregnancy journey, as it allows your growing child to receive the calcium that it needs. This calcium can be found in yogurt and milk. A deficiency in you will cause a deficiency in your unborn child, leading to health issues for you post-pregnancy. If you don't fancy yourself a great chef you can easily incorporate these ingredients into an easy smoothie. A great addition to your diet can also come in the form of daily supplements. This is helpful since all the meals we consume do not always include all the vitamins and minerals we need. Daily supplements are an easy way to increase your iron and omega 3 fatty acids (Masters, 2018).

I touched on this briefly earlier, but it's important to understand the effect that alcohol, smoking and caffeine have on your fertility as well as your partner's. Alcohol consumption has been found to negatively affect a woman's fertility. It is often unclear to what extent, but it reduces your chances of falling pregnant. Your partner's sperm count, as well as quality, is negatively affected by alcohol. The recommendation is that men consume no more than four units of alcohol a day. This might seem like a huge adjustment for your partner but it's helpful if you explain the importance that his adjustment is in your journey. A beer now and again is acceptable, so I'm sure your partner will be relieved to hear that he does not have to go completely cold turkey. Smoking is another habit that negatively impacts fertility. This one might be harder to give up for you and your partner if you both are active smokers. Smoking negatively impacts men by causing them to produce fewer sperm (DeNoon, 2010). It takes men three months to produce new sperm so preparation is key when planning for your future. It is important to start trying to conceive a child after three months of consistent healthy behavior. It also impacts your health by decreasing your chances of falling pregnant in a few ways. The main changes are in your hormone levels, the genetic makeup of your eggs, as well as slowing down your egg's ability to reach your ovary. Smoking is also harmful, not only if you are the one smoking, but through passive smoking. Passive smoking refers to the smoke you inhale by being around people who smoke. You might want to consider changing the places you frequent for a few months to improve your health. That smokey pub you enjoy going to after work on Fridays might not be the best idea anymore. This does not mean that you need to stop being social but that you must be mindful of your surroundings.

Additionally, your mental health is an important component in your pregnancy journey. I strongly encourage you to mentally prepare yourself prior to conception. This preparation time allows you to set your expectations and fears surrounding pregnancy. If you are unable to afford a professional therapist, then have an open conversation with your partner. Talking about your pregnancy journey is essential as it makes you aware of the commitment that you are making. I once heard someone describe having children as dying your hair a crazy color. You can't run away from your decision and you can't hide it from those around you. Children are a lifelong commitment, which is why it's essential that you think your decision through. This isn't meant to worry you, but just to reinforce the importance of your decision. Children might feel like dying your hair a crazy color at times but it's a fulfilling journey. It is guaranteed to be an eventful journey, but I know that it will bring you indescribable amounts of joy. It's important to remember that your children are people of their own and your job is to allow them to grow into the person they are meant to be. You are there to encourage and provide a strong support system for your children. Prenatal counselling allows you to discuss the changes that might occur in your body. It will encourage you to accept yourself in all your forms. Your mental health should be a priority throughout your journey. You need to know what your triggers are and have strategies that allow you to effectively work through your issues. These strategies will be useful to you throughout your pregnancy as well as afterwards (Green, 2018). Therapy allows you to explore your innermost feelings and work through any childhood traumas you may not be conscious of. Motherhood is a complex journey that is why preparation is key. Confronting your childhood traumas allows you to not repeat the mistakes that your parents might have made with you. It also enables you to be more understanding as you unpack the realities of parenting.

LET'S TALK ABOUT THE DOCTOR

Your doctor plays a vital role throughout your pregnancy journey. You need to have a doctor that you are comfortable with and that you trust. This is vital because you need to be able to ask questions freely without the fear of looking silly. First-time mothers are understandably bound to have many questions about pregnancy. Fertility is a word that you will need to quickly get comfortable with. It refers to your ability to produce children (Merriam-Webster, 2020). This word can seem scary at first, especially if you are actively trying to fall pregnant. It shouldn't be something to be fearful of because knowledge is power; once you know the details of your fertility, you are able to adjust your behavior to better suit your situation. You can easily test when you are most fertile through an at-home test that you can purchase at your local drug store. The test is commonly a small stick that you urinate on and it will tell you on what days you have a higher chance of falling pregnant. This simple at-home test can assist in better understanding your fertility by informing you of when you are ovulating. It is important to book an appointment with your regular gynaecologist for an examination. They are likely to check the production of your eggs as well as your fallopian tubes and uterus for any irregularities. This information will allow the doctor to make a definitive decision about the steps you need to take in order to conceive. Your gynaecologist is likely to instruct you to stop any form of contraception that you were previously using such as taking the pill, remove your IUD or to stop using the patch.

The best-case scenario is that your doctor tells you that all is well and you can conceive naturally without any medical intervention. This simply means that you and your partner can stop using all forms of contraception in the hopes of conceiving a child. If you are trying to concieve naturally, the best time to have sex is ideally in the morning. It is important to not make this too much of a routine remember trying to conceive a child should not feel like a second job. This is not the case for all women so you need to understand your options on your journey.

Hormone therapy is a common treatment option where the prospective mother is given estrogen or progesterone to assist her fertility. These hormones are useful because they directly impact your menstruation cycle, uterus and an egg's ability to attach to your uterine wall after fertilization. The hormones allow your body to make adjustments that make conception an easier process. This is a favourable treatment because it uses hormones that are naturally found in your body. This alleviates the risk involved with increasing your hormone levels. The patient is less likely to experience dangerous side effects as well as cause harm to their bodies. The treatment, as with anything you put into your body, is not without any side effects (University of Utah Health Staff, 2019). The hormones are administered through an injection or tablet. The treatment can amplify the symptoms you would commonly experience throughout your menstrual cycle such as bloating and mood swings.

In vitro fertilization (IVF) is another method that has gained popularity over the years. It is the cause of many couples who have had sextuplets or octuples. This process is commonly more expensive as it involves several more steps as compared to hormone therapy. Mature eggs need to be collected from the woman, and this is only possible through egg retrieval surgery. Preparation for the surgery involves daily hormonal injections that ensure that as many eggs as possible are mature on the day of surgery. Your partner will then be combined with your mature egg and placed in your uterus. If the procedure is effective then the embryo will attach to the uterine wall and you will officially be expecting a child. The same process can be completed with a donor egg and donor sperm. Another form of this procedure is referred to as intrauterine insemination, where sperm is directly placed into your uterus to assist it in reaching an egg. The risks of IVF is the possibility of having multiple children at one time. This is something that you need to seriously consider, because you might have only planned for one child but you are pregnant with multiple. The children are also more likely to be born before their term is over (Mayo Clinic Staff, 2019).

Miscarriages are a common occurrence during pregnancy as well as in the IVF process. A miscarriage is when your embryo detaches from the wall of your uterus. It commonly occurs within the first 3 months of pregnancy. The causes of miscarriages are still unknown but it is important to remember that normal day to day occurrences do not lead to miscarriages. It is important to take care of yourself during this time as your body is going through many changes. The symptoms that women feel in the first three months of pregnancy vary from person to person. There are women who describe the symptoms as unbearable, while others experience very minor changes. I will go into further detail about what you can expect from the first three months in more detail when we discuss labor and the different stages of pregnancy (Planned Parenthood, 2019).

Surrogacy is another option that has gained popularity in recent years with mothers assisting their daughters by offering their wombs to carry their grandchildren and long time friends taking their friendships to new heights by carrying their children. The idea of hiring another person to carry your biological child for you can be scary. This is why it's highly advised that you work with a reputable agency and hire someone that you trust. It is not a decision to take lightly because this person will be a large part of your life throughout the pregnancy journey. There are two common forms of surrogacy. The first one is referred to as traditional surrogacy in this process where sperm is inserted into the surrogate causing fertilization to occur. Genetically the child's mother is the surrogate and the father is the sperm donor. This does not mean that the child will be raised by the surrogate mother. Gestational surrogacy is far more common, as through the IVF process the child biologically belongs to the owner of the egg and sperm. The egg would belong to the mother and the sperm would come from the father. This would allow the surrogate to simply be the vessel that carries the child (Taylor, 2011). This is a helpful alternative for women who are unable to carry their children. The selection process is important as you will decide who will be a part of this journey with you. You need to consider the mental state of the applicant as well as their background. A contract is necessary between you and the surrogate to agree to payment, what the expectations are of both parties and it needs to be clearly stated that the surrogate does not have any legal claims to the child. This last clause is particularly important in areas where the law states that the individual who gives birth to the child is the legal mother.

The final alternative I will discuss is adoption. Adoption is a process where you legally become the parent of a child who was abandoned by their parents or legally placed in the foster care system because they did not have a caregiver. Adoption is beneficial as it allows you to adopt a child who already needs a home. It is beneficial to women who are past their reproductive years or people who might have prioritized their careers as opposed to childbearing. There are different options for adoption such as open and closed adoptions. Open adoptions allow for some form of communication between the biological parents and the adoptive parents. This can be through sending a photograph annually showing the biological parent the changes that have occurred in the child over the year. The communication can also be through letters or occasionally phone calls. This allows the adopted child to have an open line of communication so that there are no unanswered questions. It's helpful because adoptive children often struggle with issues of identity and belonging. The likelihood of this occurring is less frequent if the child knows where they come from. Closed adoptions, on the other hand, state that the biological parents can have no form of communication with the adoptive child. Parents are likely to select this option as it allows for more privacy. The adoption process is not easy and it can be costly, depending on where you live, so it's important to consider this when choosing to adopt. The key is to be open and understanding of the process as well as of the child you adopt (Rivard, 2017).

CHAPTER 2: WHO IS IN YOUR CORNER?

A strong support system will take you very far in this process. It's vital to know who you have around you and what role everyone will play throughout your journey. It's important to get your metaphoric house in order as well as your physical home. This is the part where honesty amongst those closest to you isn't just encouraged but it is expected. I will start with the conversation that you need to be having with your partner. Your mindset and outlook, as well as that of your partner, is what your child will be raised around. Earlier, I focused on getting your mind right but now it's important to have open conversations with your partner. The point is to create an open dialogue where both parties have space to be honest with one another and feel heard without judgment. A simple activity you can do is drawing up two lists. The first list should be about everything you are excited about when it comes to your future pregnancy and on the other side, write down all your worries. Once you have completed this task, compare your two lists and let them be a springboard to initiate a conversation with your partner. It's also extremely helpful to discuss what parenting styles you both believe in, and how you wish to raise your children. It is far easier to have an open conversation prior to the birth of your children as opposed to an argument later on in life. You need to see where you both stand when it comes to important issues like discipline, schooling or religion. Your partner should feel comfortable discussing their childhood traumas with you so that they do not repeat the mistakes of their parents. You both need to adjust your mindsets and plan around your children. You both need to have goals that match up, as it will make the transition smoother.

All the planning in the world can go a long way but you need to be practical. The truth that will ensure your survival is that you both cannot plan out what your reaction to parenthood will be. It is important to not rush one another, you need to be understanding and present, for not only the baby, but also for one another. I know that you've probably been told several times that parenting is like a switch that will instantly turn on once you lay eyes on your child. While this is true for some, it might not be for you. Be patient with your partner as well as yourself, because one person might find the switch sooner than the other. It's important to remain honest about how you feel even after the baby is born. Marriages are commonly negatively affected by the birth of children. Communication is necessary and it's easier to continue if you developed open lines of communication before conception. A study by popular baby brand Munchkin found that first-time mothers will often open up to those closest to them about any feelings of anxiety, fear or uncertainty regarding their newfound role. This is why you need to have trusted friends or relatives who you know can support you. The same support is necessary for your partner's mental health.

Important factors that I believe are not discussed often enough is preparing your finances for childbearing. The cost of a baby is affected by many factors, like the cost of necessary baby supplies or schooling. You need to decide what kind of lifestyle you hope to give your child. You need to consider the country you live in, as some are cheaper to raise children in than others. This will assist you in planning accordingly and creating a comprehensive budget. You should analyze your current monthly expenses and see what your monthly expenses are and where you can save money. It's important to estimate what your monthly expenses might look like once you have a child. This means budgeting for things like formula, clothing, hospital bills and diapers. This information will allow you to see whether your current income can accommodate a child. Your answer to this question will indicate how much saving you need to do before your child arrives. It's important to have savings regardless of how financially sound you are. Children can come with many unexpected costs and having savings will alleviate any additional stress you may develop (Salgado, 2016). It's advised that you open an investment account in your child's name to cover the cost of education or a fund in the event that something happens to you or your part-

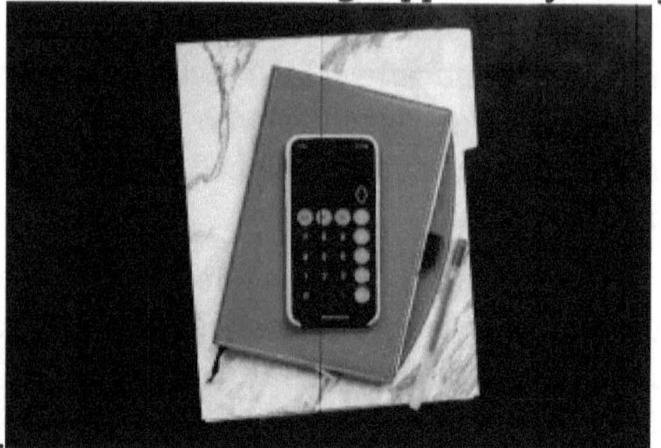

ner.

Budgeting doesn't have to be a boring activity, make a game out of it by alternating with your partner and guessing how much your monthly expenses amount to. All you need is a calculator, a piece of paper and a positive attitude. This game is only enjoyable if you are both comfortable discussing your finances and if you are both not coming from a place of judgement but rather a space of transparency. It's also important to be honest about your debts when discussing budgeting. This is a necessary skill that you should both learn, as transparency will be essential as you parent with one another. Finances can lead to increased conflict in a relationship that can lead to relationships ending. You need to look at what both your "money personalities" are. Do you enjoy spending or saving? There is no right or wrong answer to this question; you just need to be self-aware. It can be a very positive thing if both parties have different money personalities. It will allow you to balance one another out and find a middle ground between your spending habits. We should all develop healthy spending habits and encourage ourselves to save on whatever we can. Excessive spending and saving can both be detrimental (McWhinney, 2020). Developing good habits is essential as you will be able to teach your children good spending patterns.

The role that power plays concerning money in creating inequality within a relationship. You need to remain cognizant of this possibility within your relationship. Inequality can occur for many reasons such as unequal salaries, sudden unemployment or generational wealth. When money is used as a means of control it is considered a form of abuse. You need to accept your partner's financial situation and not use money to dominate or manipulate. I know that we live in a society that is continuously evolving with regard to gender roles and norms. This is an extremely positive change, so allow yourself to change with the times. Gone are the days where you just need to be a stay at home mother or worry about making more money than your partner. You can have a successful relationship even if you have unequal incomes, if there is mutual acceptance and respect.

Future mommies, make sure that you fully understand your company's maternity leave policy and when you are expected to return to work. This will allow you to plan effectively and budget around any money you may be receiving in your absence. Your partner should look into their company's paternity leave policies to see how much time they are able to spend with you after the baby is born. This allows for stay at home fathers to effectively plan while some moms go back to work. This is common for families where the mothers are the breadwinners. Financial planning also involves understanding what your health insurance covers and what you will possibly have to pay out of pocket depending on the type of delivery you would like to have. I strongly urge you to have some form of healthcare coverage regardless of the type of delivery you have, because it provides you with a sense of peace knowing that if anything were to happen and if there are any health issues with you or your child there is an effective plan in place. Planning is a key aspect of getting the people who are in your corner to all be on the same page. An effective plan adds structure and a sense of routine during your journey. This leads to decreased stress levels and increases your chances of a healthy pregnancy.

My pro tip is to draw up a will as soon as your child is born that states what would happen in the event that you or your partner are no longer available. This might seem like a grim thing to have to think about, but it's a sign of love that you have a clear plan in place for your family. You need to consult the parties that you hope will take care of your children in the event of a tragedy.

CHAPTER 3: LABOR: DECISION TIME

It's about that time where you need to make major decisions about your birthing journey. You have conceived your child and you are healthily and happily moving through all the stages. These stages are divided into three trimesters. I will briefly tell you what you need to know about each exciting stage.

The first trimester is made up from the moment of conception until week 12. This early stage of pregnancy is and where all major changes occur. Fertilization occurs when a sperm cell reaches an egg and penetrates it. This penetration changes the makeup of the egg causing it to create a barrier around it that prevents other sperm cells from entering it. The fertilized egg then attaches to the uterine wall and begins the developmental process. The heart develops and begins to beat from the sixth week onward, and the limbs begin to develop and take shape. The child's face develops and noticeable changes start to emerge in the woman's body such as fuller breasts and the dreaded morning sickness that I'm sure you've already heard about. You can also expect increased mood swings as well as heartburn. The embryo begins to look more human-like. The major organs have fully developed, and the embryo continues to grow. Things like the human skeleton, genitals, eyes and ears form (Stanway, 2000). You can begin to make shifts to your daily routine to allow for new changes. The child begins to develop the formation of the major organs, as well as the nervous system. You are most at risk of a miscarriage during this time, as there are many changes occurring in your body. If you experience any bleeding, seek medical attention immediately.

The second trimester is from week 13 through to 28 the chances of a miscarrying are less likely than in the first trimester. Your child is still quite small but many of the organs begin to function. This includes a mock breathing function. The fingers and toes begin to develop and other small details like eyelashes also form. The child continues to freely move around as they are protected by a vernix that takes care of the baby's skin. The 19th week onward, the child has likely grown to 30cm and continues to develop and move. Your child will begin to notice outside stimuli such as instrumentals and voices. You are likely to be "showing" during this time as a clear baby bump develops. Week 25 through to 28 come with exciting changes for mommy and baby as your child's eyes open. Your child can experience hiccups and suck their thumb. You can also begin to experience practice contractions as you are nearing your delivery date (Stanway, 2000).

The third and final trimester is from week 29 through to 40 during this time some children are born and are likely to survive. Your baby is still kicking and moving even if it is starting to feel a little cramped. You can identify the different body parts as they poke and prod you. Your child has put on a considerable amount of weight and likely weighs about 2.4 kilograms/5 pounds. In week 33 onwards your child should move into the head-down position in preparation for labor. It's important to remember that your due date is an estimate of when you are expected to give birth. You need to mentally prepare yourself that your child could come a few weeks sooner or a few weeks later. Mental strength will carry you through this time. Remember that pregnancy is a natural process that many have gone through before you and you to have the strength to endure it.

Your health comes first, now more than ever because you directly impact your child. Regular doctor visits are mandatory to track the development of your child. In these visits, you will be able to ask any questions that you may have and discuss the changes that are happening to your body. Most importantly, you will get your first chance to see your child for many women this moment solidifies the start of their journey. The same can be said for your partner who is not carrying the child. Scans are vital because they allow you to monitor the growth of your child and hear their heartbeat. This moment can lead to a little surprise for some parents as they discover that they are having more than one child. There are medical issues that can commonly arise during pregnancy such as chronic headaches. It is important to monitor your symptoms so that your doctor can correctly treat you throughout your pregnancy. Your doctor will also advise you on the correct vitamins and minerals to take, as well as further information on your diet and exercise. You will quickly learn that adaptation is vital as your body continues to change. Your exercise routine will need to adapt as your tummy continues to grow because your level of mobility begins to change.

It's now time to discuss one of the most important decisions that you will make regarding your pregnancy. How do you plan on welcoming your child into the world? Thankfully, there are many options to choose from, so you are able to select the one that best suits you. I will start by discussing the most popular option which is natural childbirth. This process is widely recommended by midwives and nurses as it usually leads to a quicker and smoother recovery process. This process occurs naturally when the gestation period is over. Your cervix will begin to soften and you will notice a clear gel-like liquid similar to discharge. This is known as your mucus plug, your water will likely break and your labor process begins. You will begin to experience contractions, it is vital that you monitor the duration of the contractions and duration of the intervals. The closer the intervals indicates the speed of your labor. Your cervix will begin to dilate as it prepares for labor.

You are now in early labor until your cervix reaches 3cm. The process begins to move at a quicker pace from this point on as you move from 3cm through to 7cm this phase is known as active labor. Regardless of whether you are in a hospital or giving birth in your home with a midwife,the professional will closely monitor your heart rate and movement. You are ready to start pushing when you are at a full 10cm. These phases are all marked by different symptoms such as lower back pain and increased pain levels through your contraction. Water consumption, as well as mental strength is essential in this time because you need to make sure that you do not panic and stay calm. The natural labor process is now fully underway and you will begin to push your child out of your vaginal canal. Once the child has entered the world, the doctor will cut the umbilical cord connecting the child to the mother. In some instances, your partner has the opportunity to cut the umbilical cord. In addition to this, there are variations that you can make to the natural birth process. One of these alterations that are commonly used is the use of pain relief medication. This is commonly in the form of an injection in your lower spine. It relieves all the pain associated with birth. This drug can only be administered in a hospital setting. There are less invasive drugs that alleviate other symptoms of birth. They commonly handle nausea or disorientation. Natural labor is recommended as the recovery process is usually quicker and easier.

Another alternative is the use of a midwife; midwives

are not new as they have been used for many generations. I briefly mentioned midwives earlier, and now I will go into further detail. A midwife is a trained professional who delivers your child in the comfort of your own home or at a registered birthing centre. This option is often preferred by mothers who are not fond of hospitals or conventional medicine. This option is often cheaper than hospitalization, and mothers are commonly more satisfied with the service they received as opposed to other methods. This is suitable because midwives are registered professionals, so be sure to do your research and use a trusted known professional. The midwife will provide all the necessary equipment for the labor process.

Waterbirth has grown in popularity over the years with more and more mothers giving it a try. It is commonly performed in a birthing centre or your home by a registered midwife. You will be in a warm bath during labor, this method is promoted by many mothers as a more natural alternative. It's considered more natural because your child has been in amniotic fluid throughout your pregnancy so delivering in water is considered less of a shock for the baby. Women express that water helps with some pain relief and alleviates stress. Waterbirth can come with some risks such as infection from anything that you expel during the process. You might pass some feces during this process and it's nothing to be ashamed about because it's a natural process. There is the worry of your child drowning but this is very uncommon as the medical professional assisting you ensures that the child is not underwater for an extended period of time (Besich & Hochwald, 2020). There isn't a blueprint to giving birth naturally as every woman's experiences are different.

A popular option for women who would like to give birth in a hospital is a cesarean section. A cesarean section is a surgery that allows you to surgically deliver your child. This process is quick and very well planned. You are given a general anaesthetic that allows you to be numb but awake during the procedure. This lets you speak to your partner throughout the procedure and communicate with the doctors and nurses. Out of view from you, the doctor will cut across your lower uterus and expose your child. Your child will be removed from you immediately, cleaned and suctioned to remove any fluid from the lungs. This is an option recommended for women who are carrying multiple children or those who have a child that is unable to turn into the birthing position. It is also advised for women who are infected with HIV, as it decreases the chances of transferring it to their newborn child. It is a preferred choice if you opt not to give birth through your vaginal canal. It is important to consider many factors when deciding on this option such as the mother's age, medical history, weight and any other complications related to the pregnancy. If these complications are not correctly handled, they can be dangerous for you and your baby. That may be your intended delivery option, but complications can arise during this process. This can occur if your labor process is taking too much time and the mother or child begin to get tired. A drop in the heart rate of the mother or child also means that an operation is needed. It is nothing to be fearful of as the operation has become a very common procedure. This process allows women the freedom of choice in many ways, as many worry about their recovery process. You have the opportunity to select your childbirth date and select a period that is convenient for you. Plus, there is the added benefit of not having to worry about labor pains during the process. The recovery process is more extensive than that of natural labor as you are recovering from surgery. You will require more assistance and days in the hospital after the procedure.

All of these different options for delivery offer you the beauty of choice and your choice is the most important factor. You need to know what you want your delivery experience to be and what your plan b is in case there are complications. It is important to put your health, as well as the health of your child, first. You both must receive the best possible treatment regardless of if it's from a doctor or a midwife. The Baby Centre Medical Advisory Board (2020) found a breathing technique that you can use through most of these options called controlled breathing. This technique can be very effective in calming both mommy and their partner down. It is about using all of your energy to focus on your breathing, as opposed to your contractions. You can do this by picking any word to focus on, I suggest a word that brings you joy like love, positivity, strength or conqueror. I suggest a word that makes you feel empowered that will allow you to channel all of your emotions into that word. Simply start by thinking of the word you have chosen and sync your breathing to that word. Inhale on the first part of the word and exhale on the second. Allow yourself to get lost in the word and let it bring you a sense of control. This is important because the labor process can feel as though it's out of your control. You need to remain calm and composed. Your partner can help alleviate any stress you may be experiencing by reassuring you and assisting you through your breathing exercises.

CHAPTER 4: IT'S THE BIG DAY!

I have titled this chapter *The Big Day!* because that's what holding your child in your arms for the first time feels like. Once your child is in your arms, for many people it feels like a long-awaited prize that you have dreamed and hoped for. It is a moment that is so euphoric that it is somewhat indescribable. You are now officially a mommy, and while this can feel scary, it's an exciting moment and experience. I know this moment can feel overwhelming, but I'll give you some clear steps on what to do next. It is always helpful to have a plan in place.

In preparation for the big day, it's important to have a few things in place. We will start by talking about how to book a room for your birth, and what to pack in your hospital bag. You can confidently say what your birthing plan is and where you would like to give birth, whether this is at a hospital, birthing centre or in your home, some preparations are needed to be made for the day. Your monthly visits to the doctor for your ultrasounds will inform you of your expected delivery date.

Your hospital or centre should have a copy of your health insurance information and clearly state what is included and what will come out of pocket. In the case of a caesarian section, your birth is planned down to the minute, which gives some moms peace of mind as they can plan around it. Discuss with your doctor what day you would prefer, and make an appointment. If you have decided to give birth naturally, then your birth is planned in a specific window. Your doctor will have a room ready for you and the birthing centre will do the same. In the case of a midwife, the person will come over to your home once you give them the call that you are in labor.

If you are anything like me, you are probably lost about what you need and maybe buying too many of the same things. Luckily a hospital bag is something that you have time to plan for. Your hospital bag should have a few necessary things. I will go through what should be in your bag and what you should put in your partner's bag. It might be surprising but your partner also needs to have a few supplies. I will go through what should be in your partner's bag first. The first thing you should have stored away in a file are copies of your identity documentation and health insurance. It is ideal to take the originals with you on the day of, but this allows you to have a backup in case you forget your originals on the big day. Your partner should have a few snacks packed so that no one needs to leave the room if anyone gets hungry. It's hard to estimate how long your labor will be, so it's important to prepare for all possible scenarios. I know we've all experienced that moment where we realize that we left the house without charging our phones. Don't let that be you on the day of delivery, ensure that your phone is sufficiently charged and that you have packed a charger and power bank. This will give you peace of mind by allowing you to communicate with your relatives or close loved ones who are not at the hospital with you. You will also be able to document the labor process for future memories through pictures and videos. Parents will often make a short video speaking to their future daughter or son before birth, and stating how they feel at that moment. This is a sweet memory that will be a timeless gift from your child. A quick pro-tip would be to remember to back all of this up on an online cloud as soon as you can, because these are precious moments that you don't want to lose. There are many online free clouds that you can use. It is important to pack a change of clothes in case there are any accidents for you and your partner. You need to be comfortable during the process and ensure that your partner is positive and in good spirits. It's important to pack a few activities for you two to play while you wait. This can be novels, playing cards, magazines or crossword puzzles. You need to have these options available even if your partner decides not to use them.

The hospital bag is filled with supplies that are geared toward the mother after she has given birth. The facility you give birth in might offer a few supplies, so take this into consideration when you pack your bag. The must-have items consist of a change of clothes for the new mom, underwear, nursing pads, pregnancy pads, slippers and toiletries. It's important to have clothing that is loose and comfortable because trust me the last thing you will want is a tight pair of pants on. A few pairs of comfortable underwear that are cotton for less irritation are vital. This isn't the time to break out your favourite lace set. A comfortable maternity bra is a necessity as well as absorbent nursing pads. They will ensure that you don't have any unexpected leaking. Pregnancy pads are important because you will experience heavy bleeding after labor, and pads cause less irritation and lower the chances of an infection. Slippers are a staple because you will want a comfortable pair of shoes to wear around your hospital room. General toiletries like a face cloth, toothpaste, soap and body lotion will come in handy as you stay at the hospital for a few days (Kashtan, 2019). Your new baby will need a first outfit. I know a few moms who take this very seriously as it's the first outfit their child will wear. It will also appear in all the early photos. You don't have to stress yourself out about this. A comfortable onesie is perfectly adequate. If you do not intend on breastfeeding, a few bottles are also necessary. Your time in the hospital is intended for your recovery, but resting in a bed all day isn't for everyone, so use this time to rest and enjoy yourself. Your child will be by your side so this allows you time to begin to bond. An essential must-have when leaving the hospital is a car seat so that your baby is comfortable and well-protected. This is a requirement if you are leaving a hospital with a newborn child.

NAMING

One of the most important decisions that I believe can come about during your pregnancy and motherhood journey is naming your child. The exciting yet somewhat scary question of, "What should I name my child?" I believe it was Shakespeare who said that *"a rose by any other name would still smell as sweet"*, now I'm not trying to make this a high school English lesson, but if we take this statement into account, your child's name isn't that important. If we follow this logic, your child will still turn out to be the person who they are intended to be. Naming your child is an opportunity to decide how you would like to introduce your child into the world. It's the first thing that many people will hear, and a name that you will say more times than you can count. It would be wise to choose a name that you actually like and feel comfortable with. It's also important to consider what the different nickname options might be for your child because the schooling system isn't the nicest to children who are different. This doesn't mean that you should be fearful of what you name your child because regardless of what you name your child, you will teach them self-awareness and self-love. If you follow any celebrity news then you know that they are notorious for giving their children weird and mildly peculiar names. We have heard names like Apple, Blue, North or even a series of symbols in some cases. This is alright if you are the child of a celebrity, because their lives were never really normal to begin with but for the everyday person, these names are a little harder to swallow. I know that parents are tired of being conventional by choosing names that have been around for decades. Naming is a way of ensuring individuality for your child, so remember to pick a name that speaks to you as opposed to simply following trends.

A study by the authors of *Freakonomics* found that the name you give your child can shape the person that they become. You want your child to embody the name that you give them. Think about, your name is the the first gift you recieve when you come into the world and the last thing people remember when you ar gone. So strive for a name with a solid meaning or one that has sentimental value. This can be a family name passed down for many generations for some parents, or a completely new name that they hope their child grows into or acquires strength from. It can be hard to decide what to name your child because you have never met them and understandably many parents would prefer to know what their child's nature and personality is like before naming them. This is not entirely possible because in some areas your child is required to have a name in order to leave the hospital. It is advised that you understand the laws of your area so you know how much time you have. In some areas, you have a few days and in others, you can have up to a year. In some places, children are required to have a name before they depart from the hospital (Magher, 2017). I would advise that you not take too much time to decide on this because that last thing you want to procrastinate over is the name of your child. It can lead to delays in the documentation and unnecessary penalty fees. A name also helps with the bonding process with your baby, so the sooner you can name them the better; with some moms deciding during their pregnancy. When you first start thinking about baby names, you can draw up a list of names you have always loved. Your partner can do the same thing and you can take turns making suggestions on what you believe are the best options. This list will help you in deciding once your child has arrived. This can be a great bonding activity for both of you because it allows you to think about your future. There are many online resources that have baby name suggestions and rank the popularity of each name for you. The search for a perfect baby name can be extended to your close friends and family if you need a little more help. What I am sure of is that at the end of the day, the name you give your child will be perfect for you, the child and your family. A quick pro-tip if you are struggling to decide between two names for your child: Give your child both names. Depending on the child, a middle name can provide them with an option of what they would like to be called. Nicknames are also extremely helpful and convenient for both mommy and baby. Parents can develop special names for their children that become a staple in their relationship. If the unexpected happens and your child completely hates their name as they grow up, simply sit them down and explain why you selected it. This small gesture will allow your child to understand what your thought-process was and know that you cared about them.

Support is a topic that I have spoken about before, but it's important to remember that it's a vital component in every stage and that the support you are given changes with the stage that you are in. Support during your birth process is likely to come from your partner and the medical professionals around you. Your partner must be in tune with you and compassionate about what you are experiencing. They should remember the skills that they acquired in counselling. Your family and friends will begin to trail in to visit you after the birth of the child. It is important to be present in the moment and not worry about your appearance or clothing too much. They are all there to offer you love and support, not to judge your appearance. There's the excitement to meet the new addition into your life as well as theirs. The visits will give you time to rest as well while your visitors look after your child. If you are not in the position to have any relatives or friends visit you, remember that the nurses and staff are there to support you. You can speak to them and ask any questions you may have. A friendly relationship allows you to be comfortable enough to bring up any concerns or medical issues you may be experiencing.

Preparing your home for the arrival of a child can seem overwhelming but I believe it should be an enjoyable process that allows for creativity. If you live in a home that allows your child to have their own bedroom, then a nursery is a fantastic idea from the beginning. If you do not have this luxury, or you would prefer your child in your room for the first few years, in a crib then that is also acceptable. No matter the situation, your child will need things that you probably do not already have in your home. You will need a crib, like this one, for your child. There are a large variety of options available in different price ranges to suit your budget. This crib will need a set of bedding. I suggest selecting a soft breathable material that is easily washable. A mobile above the child crib is a great source of stimulation because they come in a variety of shapes and colours that will be eye-catching to your new baby. The positioning of the crib should be in a neutral area where the child is not in direct contact with either an air conditioning system or direct sunlight. A comfortable resting chair is a great investment because you will be spending many hours seated in this room. A changing table and changing mat are essential and a necessity especially in the first few months when your child is using a large number of diapers. A diaper bin is also a must-have item for any nursery. Storage, you will soon learn, is something that you can never have enough of as your child begins to grow.

A dresser or a full wardrobe in the room will be beneficial to store all the bits and bobs you never seem to have space for. Your storage should be easily accessible to you and the order allows you to form a routine. It is important that you like your child's nursery because you will be spending many hours there in the first few months. The flooring in the room should be comfortable, and a designated play area for the child is a great addition. A playmat is a great alternative if you do not have a lot of space in your home. The playmat will be suitable for your child's tummy time and it gives them an area to learn how to crawl. Books are a great addition because it allows you to speak to your child and form a routine. The most important thing you can have is a baby monitor. It will give you peace of mind and allow you to be busy around the house without having to worry about how your baby is doing. New moms are often worried about their child's breathing and their comfort level while they sleep. The advancements in baby monitors let you virtually be in the room with your child; this is also a great tool for the parent who is not at home all day because it allows them to check in on the baby now and again (Braaksma, n.d.). Here are a few ideas for decorating your baby's room:

I know that with the increase in popularity of social media accounts and all of us getting a sneak peek at how celebrities decorate their kid's rooms, it can be hard to decide what you want your unique style to be. The key factors to consider are creating a room that is child-friendly and that you can easily adapt to as the child grows up. In the early days, your child is adjusting to a new environment, so it's helpful to create a space that is simple and comfortable. There is a growing trend for children's rooms to be more monochromatic and include less color, but it's important to remember that your child's development is influenced by their environment. Color acts as an effective stimulant for your child. Have fun with colors as you decorate and include different textures for your child to experience. The color can be through the furniture, toys, bedding or the use of paintings on a wall. These types of pops of color are easily changeable as the child grows up and develops their style and interests. Different changes will need to be made to your home as your child grows, like security gates and outlet protectors. The decoration of the nursery is your time to introduce your child to different things and peak their interests in

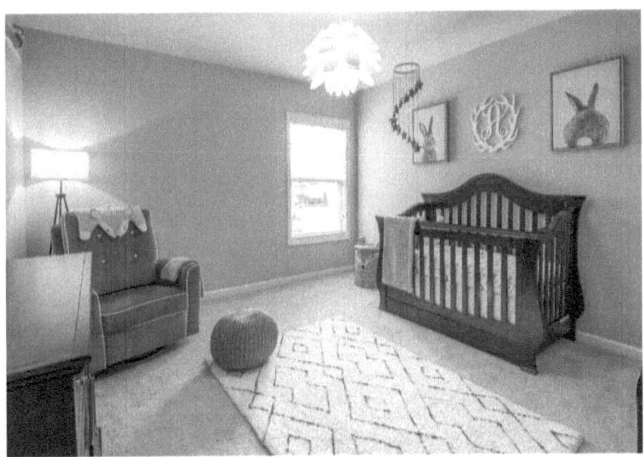

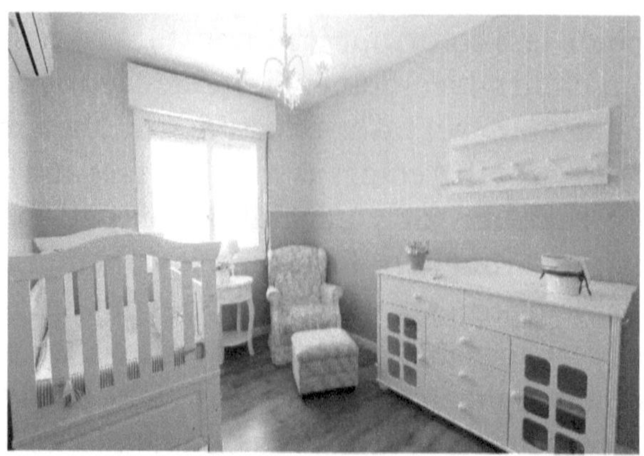

topics that will shape how they view the world.

CHAPTER 5: CHILDBIRTH AFTERMATH:

What's in Store for Me?

Recovery is just as important as preparation. Once you have given birth, depending on the method you have selected, you will experience different immediate reactions. If natural birth was your choice then you are required to expel your placenta after giving birth. This starts the process of your body's natural cleansing process. You are obviously tired and will need to rest for a short time as your body has gone through many new feelings during the birth process. If you surgically delivered your child then you are recovering from the anaesthesia and resting up. You will be given an area to rest and begin your recovery. Recovery may sound like an extreme word, but it simply means that it is a designated time for your body to go back to normal. This period is important as your body went through many changes.

Your health is the most important thing and you can only truly take care of your child after you take care of yourself. You need to be honest with the medical staff taking care of you and express any issues you may be experiencing. This is extremely important for women who are members of previously marginalised groups. The healthcare system has not always considered the feelings of the mother and disregarded any symptoms they might be experiencing as exaggerations. This is why it's important to be around medical professionals that you trust and can express yourself around. These health issues could be fatal and lead to death. You and your partner need to know what the warning signs are so that you can both be aware of any changes that occur in the new mom. These symptoms range from a fever, excessive pain, excessive bleeding or unusual smelling discharge. The more severe symptoms that are evident are disorientation, drastic shifts in body temperature that can be from excessive heat to extreme cold. A change in heart rate is a common sign that the new mother is experiencing a medical issue associated with childbirth. A good rule of thumb is to mention any changes you experience regardless of how tiny you think they might be. It is always better to be safe than sorry especially when it comes to your health.

The common health issues that could arise after birth range from heart issues to postpartum depression. Postpartum depression is very common amongst many women who do not receive adequate support after the birth of their child (Corrigan, et al., 2015). I remember a few months after I had given birth to my first child that I experienced feelings of being overwhelmed and a continual feeling of being lost. I was often extremely sad and lacked any real motivation. I then realized that I was simply going through the motions and trying my best to take care of my son. It was at this time that I began to have more and more arguments with my partner over tiny disagreements. I did not feel any support from my partner while my partner believed that he was providing me with adequate support. I had always been a very self-sufficient person but raising my child was something that I felt I could not handle by myself. I decided to speak to a professional and it became clear that I was experiencing postpartum depression. Of course I was able to work through this by receiving more support from my partner and those around me. The therapist gave me the space needed to freely discuss my fears and recommended some tools to adjust. In addition, chest pains and increased heart rate are often signs of heart disease. Heart problems are a dangerous side effect for some women whose bodies do not return to their normal state. This can be a sign of blood clots forming in your body another sign is a shift in the color of your skin. This is very dangerous if these clots move towards your heart or your lungs. It can result in the loss of life of many women. Roughly 700 women pass away from complications after childbirth; vigilance can ensure that you do not fall into this category (Centers for Disease Control and Prevention, 2019).

There are less severe issues that could arise after childbirth that are not life-threatening but should be monitored. When you are aware of these possibilities, then if any of them arise you are not completely caught off guard. Stretch marks are extremely common in most women after pregnancy. They are most visible around your stomach area and thigh region. They occur around the areas where the skin stretched the most. There are many at-home remedies to help remove these stretch marks but I have found that they are not 100% effective. If they assist, then they are likely to only help lessen the visibility of the stretch marks. Tissue oils can be effective in helping your skin recover. Hair loss is another issue that could arise due to pregnancy that isn't often discussed for many women. Their hair is their pride and joy, so the thought of this can be extremely scary. The common cause of this is the shift in hormone levels in your body. Stress in new moms can also manifest itself through hair loss (Marcin, 2018). It is important to not worry yourself about this too much because it often resolves itself with time. You should not put too much strain on your hair and accept the changes.

The last unexpected issue that could arise is after childbirth is a decrease in sexual desire. Sex after pregnancy is recommended only after a full month to six weeks after giving birth. This takes into consideration the time estimated for your body to remove any mucus or blood. This recommendation is also to ensure that your body has had an adequate amount of time to heal.

When you finally try to be intimate with your partner it can be disappointing to discover that you no longer enjoy sex and that it can be extremely uncomfortable and even painful. The clinical term for it is dyspareunia; in simple terms, it means any pain that is caused by sexual activity or sexual climate. If you are experiencing this, honesty with your partner is vital as you will both be more aware of what the issues are. This knowledge allows you both to effectively find a way to resolve this. The shift in hormones can be caused by breastfeeding or a shift to regular hormone levels after pregnancy. This can lead to decreased levels of libido causing a decrease in your desire for sex. The physical changes that your body has undergone due to childbirth include pressure on your pelvic floor. This disorder is present in all forms of birth so it's important to be aware of the changes your body is experiencing. A way to effectively treat this is by seeing your gynaecologist for an examination of your body. This will show if you have any scar tissues or unknown rips. Booking an appointment with your local therapist can also be effective because it allows you an open space to express your feelings. This disorder has been associated with general relationship issues. A hormonal cream or addition of lubricants can be a great addition in alleviating pain. It is important to remember that sex is fully enjoyable when both parties are fully committed and present. It's important to be honest about your feelings. Exercises like kegels are very effective in helping strengthen your pelvic floor. This is the right time to try out new positions and new ways to pleasure one another while you are adjusting to your new body. See it as an adventure for you and your partner to try new things (Murkoff, 2018)

Your new body is something that might take a bit to get used to. Your body has been through this life-changing process where for 40 weeks of your life you were pregnant, then one day you go into labor and you are officially a mother. The only issue is that your stomach doesn't instantly deflate, so you still look pregnant. You'll continue to look pregnant for a few weeks. This truth is hard for most mothers to accept as they all want to get their old bodies back as soon as possible. There are many influences as to why women want to snap back so quickly and one of the major ones is celebrity culture. We have all seen celebrity mothers get their post-pregnancy bodies back in a matter of a few weeks. We all wonder how they have the energy to do this and how unbelievable it all seems. The truth is many celebrities undergo plastic surgery after giving birth or immediately start extreme diets. This is possible because they can afford to hire 24-hour care for their newborn. Social media also affects our expectations of how long we should rest before starting to exercise again. We see mommy influencers who all seem to have everything figured out but we don't take into consideration that a picture is just a representation of one moment. We don't consider all the tools that people use to edit their bodies to seem more favourable after giving birth.

The important thing that you need to know is that you

are not in competition with anyone so it's vital to go at your own pace. Remember that your baby needs you, so it's important to preserve your energy. Do not start exercising before you have completely healed as it can impact your healing process. It's also understandable if you don't have the energy to workout or even think about it. Your plate is understandably full, so you have to take things slow. The first step is to start with simple stretches that allow you to strengthen your body. You can find simple, easy-to-follow plans from your medical advisor or through a simple online search. You can schedule this before you start your day or before going to bed. The stretches assist in regaining flexibility and can have calming qualities. Wearing a post-pregnancy belt is strongly suggested because it gives you support and helps your body to return to its regular shape. This is effective so that when you start exercising more your back is more supported. I would suggest giving yourself nothing short of a year to regain mobility and effectively exercise. You can increase the intensity of your workout plan as you continue to get more comfortable. There isn't an instant fix to weight-loss, so remember that your fitness journey is completely reliant on you. You need to remember that your new body is the result of your new child so don't beat yourself up about it. Love yourself and accept yourself in every form. You can do this by doing small gestures for yourself. This can be through simply applying some lipstick in the morning or styling your hair. These small gestures will reinforce your confidence as you get used to your new body.

CHAPTER 6: LEAN ON ME

I'm sure you must be tired of hearing it by now, but your journey will be more enjoyable if there are people around to support you. This can be through supportive friends, co-workers or family. If you do not have anyone around you, joining a community group for single parents or parenting classes can be very helpful. These classes can be online or in-person, but it's important to have a few people around you who you can trust. A great way to adjust is through parenting classes that will help you learn how to effectively parent. There is a very popular song that talks about the importance of having someone to lean on. You are guaranteed to have moments where you will be with your new baby and feeling completely lost. In these moments, it's helpful to have some skills or a few tricks that you can pull out of your bag.

Parenting classes give you a solid foundation and practical knowledge about how to do many things. Parenting classes might feel like a lot of unneeded pressure but they are often just a safe space for all new parents to learn, and more importantly, talk. It might be the only space where you can openly say that you watch your baby sleep sometimes because you're worried that something might happen, or that you've accidentally put the diaper on the wrong way a few too many times. It is a safe space because you should be surrounded by like-minded people. When deciding on a group, it's important to look at what the group stands for and how diverse the group is. This will expose you to more diverse people and a wider variety of opinions if you ever need one. You don't ever want to be surrounded by mommy-shamers who only ever discuss how great they are at preventing. Your child is also likely to grow up with some of these people around so it is an opportunity to make a few friends. The time you have to socialise as well as the social skills that you develop can prevent the onset of depression. It is also beneficial for your baby to be around other babies as you'll watch in wonder at the way they communicate with one another. Your child's communication with other children can seem almost magical depending on the ages. It will be marked by big smiles, squeals and a lot of laughter. Your baby needs to be around other children as it helps their development. If you aren't very social then you might need to make a few adjustments to help your child developmentally and build how they interact with others.There are links to your child's confidence and verbal development. It is important to remember that from the moment your child is born they begin to start continuously learning. The classes allow your child to be exposed to new environments and people

(Vercelletto, 2018).

There are a wide variety of the types of classes that you can take with your baby such as basic parenting tutorials for everyday tasks, yoga classes that help you both with your flexibility, and massage classes that help you bond with your child. I want to highlight music classes and the benefits that they have on your child. It's a great option because it helps your child's motor skills develop, and they are able to develop emotional intelligence, cognitive development, and language development through interactions with other children. You will quickly realize what your child enjoys doing, and pick classes that suit both your needs. There are classes that are specifically suited to older children that you will have the opportunity to take as your child grows older. These include dance classes that can help with coordination, flexibility and act as a form of exercise. Art classes are another great way to spend time with your child as they grow older and continue to develop. Online classes are the easier choice for some mothers, because you can access it from the comfort of your home. While your baby is napping, you can catch up on new classes and get advice that is usually from medical experts depending on the program you are a part of. These classes help you with tips and tricks that you might not be aware of on how to effectively take care of your baby. The classes cover everything from dietary options, to bonding with your baby, to nursery decoration.

The first year of your child's life is extremely nerve-racking and exciting at the same time. You will be worried and excited by every squeal, giggle or even every diaper change. I believe that planning for your first year is extremely important and beneficial to both baby and parent. The frenzy of having a new child can often throw your life into a whirlwind. I suggest buying a planner or printing out a free template for every month of the year. This lets you plan out important dates and mark milestones when your child hits them. It gives you time to plan when you want to have photoshoots or take classes with your baby. If you are on maternity leave, you will be able to clearly see when you need to return to work and how long your income will sustain you for. Your budgeting will need to be well-planned out so that you don't find yourself overspending or in a financial slum. Planning helps alleviate stress and anxiety that is extremely common in first-time mothers. Your plan should also include when you will be seeing the doctor for your baby's monthly check-ups. This helps you never miss an appointment and stay on track. Your health can also be tracked as you begin to slowly exercise again and regain your strength. You can monitor the changes in your body by including a section for your personal developments. This helps you keep track of any issues that you might need to mention to your doctor.

Your support system is also more likely to help out with the baby if you ask them a few months in advance. This lets you go grocery shopping alone or enjoy a date night with your partner without worrying about childcare. Childcare is a huge expense for many parents, because it's difficult to find someone who you can trust with the necessary experience. This is why trusted family members are a great alternative because you know that they have good intentions and will effectively care for your child. There have been many horror stories about professional child caregivers who cause harm to the child they look after. This can be in the form of physical, emotional or sexual abuse. You need to be mindful of these possibilities because not everyone has good intentions. You can prevent this by speaking to your children as they grow older about what is right and what is wrong, as well as how adults should and should not touch them. You can spot any mistreatment if you notice any drastic changes in your child's behavior or personality. A few easy steps can be followed when looking for a caregiver, or if you're thinking of sending your child to a daycare facility. The first thing you should do is ask any other mothers around you if there is someone that they trust and read reviews about the person or facility. When you visit a facility, look at the facilities that they have for the children, the safety measures that are in place and most importantly, how the employees treat the children. It is also important to know what their values and thoughts are around discipline. The final decision is yours regardless of what they try to sell to you, so be sure to go with your instincts; if you have a bad feeling about a place, keep looking at other options regardless of how desperately you need a center. The place you decide on will have a large impact on how your child develops and the way that they behave, so do not take this decision lightly (Boardwell, 2002).

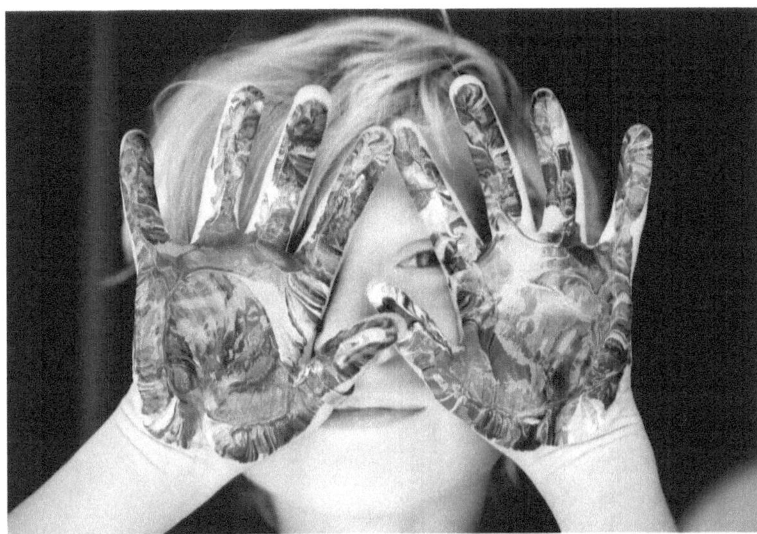

Your child's first birthday is a milestone for all parents as it symbolizes the completion of the first year of life. Parents often mark this day with a huge celebration for their child, but I think it's helpful to offer a few alternatives to the big expensive birthday party. You can plan a very small get-together to thank the people that have helped you get to this point. This can be a nice dinner or lunch at your home where it is just about spreading love. You can plan an at-home photo shoot for your baby that doesn't have to break the bank. All you need is a solid background, a costume and a few props. This is your opportunity to get creative so think outside the box. You just need to start with a theme like a pirate, sailor, princess, bunny theme or something more abstract like the rainbow, polka dots, black and white, or the galaxy. Once you have a theme, it's easier to plan around that when deciding what you'll need. A great way to get your baby to smile or laugh is to dangle their favourite toy in front of them or sing a song. Parents also enjoy recreating their baby pictures with their children (Hartshorn & Tomlin, n.d.). A great way to mark this milestone is to cast your child's handprints and footprints in a mould. This is a great memento that you can keep and show to your child later on.

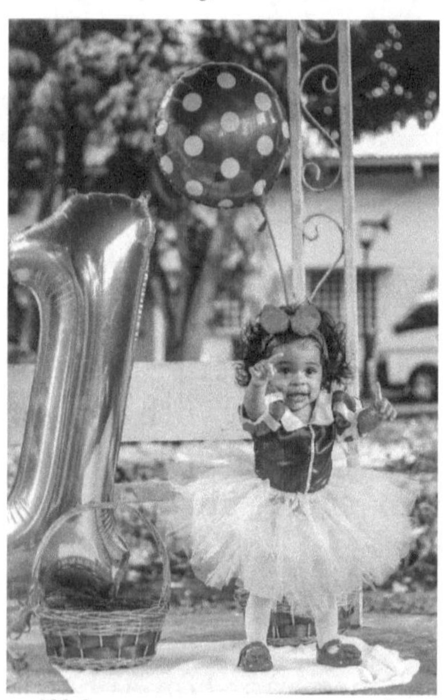

Your partner will be a great source of support for you once you have a child. The dynamic of your relationship will change once you have a child, as you both readjust your previous priorities to cater to your child. Your child will become the first thing you think about when you make major decisions. Once this change occurs, it can be hard for either of you to adjust to the new dynamic where you are no longer the priority. Your relationship needs to be able to withstand this change and this is only possible through open and honest communication. You need to make time for one another so that you do not forget about your relationship. In order to be an effective parent, you need to prioritize one another. This is through date nights, conversations during meal times or even just small moments of intimacy between the two of you. Your partner should be your biggest support system as you both navigate this new journey. We will discuss the importance of being comfortable with yourself and how that affects your relationship in a later chapter specifically dedicated to you, Mommy.

CHAPTER 7: NEWBORN:

You Officially Have a Baby

Parenthood is a complex journey that will take more than a few days to adjust yourself to. Earlier, we spoke about the importance of having frank conversations with your partner about what you both expect from one another. Now that you both have a newborn, your expectations might not be met and some adjustments will need to be made to your original plan. Newborns are completely reliant on you for their survival and the original plan that you had might not be possible or practical anymore. You need to be open to adapting your plans to better suit the situation. Your newborn needs care, love, and support. You might be struggling with how to bond with your newborn but the point of this manual is to give you a clear guide. I will explain easy to follow bonding techniques with your child and the importance of your child's positioning throughout the day.

Similarly, there are a few easy activities that you can

complete with your baby to help you both bond with one another. A well-known technique is called skin-to-skin. This is the simple task of placing your child directly on your bare chest. If there are no medical complications, then this technique is used in the first few moments after your child's birth. It is recommended because it allows your child's breathing to be synced with your heart rate. This has a calming effect on your child, and the proximity bonds the two of you together. The bonding works in many forms but especially through the physical contact with your new child that you carried for many months. I believe that it is a surreal feeling for the majority of first-time moms. It is a physical representation of many sleepless nights, nausea and an ever-growing baby bump. It lets you experience a new type of closeness with your child. This is an activity that you can add to your day to day routine to spend time with your baby. This is also beneficial for your partner who may not get to spend the entire day with the child in the early days as you do. It allows them an allocated amount of time of pure bonding. This allows the baby to get accustomed to them as well. The benefits of this activity continue to be studied and documented. There is a direct correlation with skin-to-skin and your baby's development concerning weight gain, better sleep because it has calming effects, and the regulation of your child's physiological responses specifically body temperature and heartbeat. The most substantial benefit I believe is the cognitive benefits, motor skills development and brain development. You may be skeptical about the benefits, but this is a tried and tested method that has worked for many generations.

The benefits also surpass just bonding for the parent; it allows you to develop much-needed confidence in taking care of your child. This is because when you are doing this activity, you are completely aware of your child's movements and breaths. It enables you to develop pride in your abilities and increase your nurturing instincts. These instincts are necessary because they make you more alert and in tune to your child's needs. In the relationship between mother and child, it helps make breastfeeding easier. You are likely to produce more milk and have an easier time feeding your child, subsequently increasing your confidence levels (Gebauer-Steinick, 2020). While this activity is extremely beneficial, you should be cautious of taking a nap when your child falls asleep on your chest. This can be dangerous because you are unaware of your child's positioning and breathing if they are asleep on your chest while you nap. I know that most moms try to sneak in a nap whenever their child sleeps, but it is more beneficial for you to either remove your child from your chest once they fall asleep or be wide awake while your child naps.

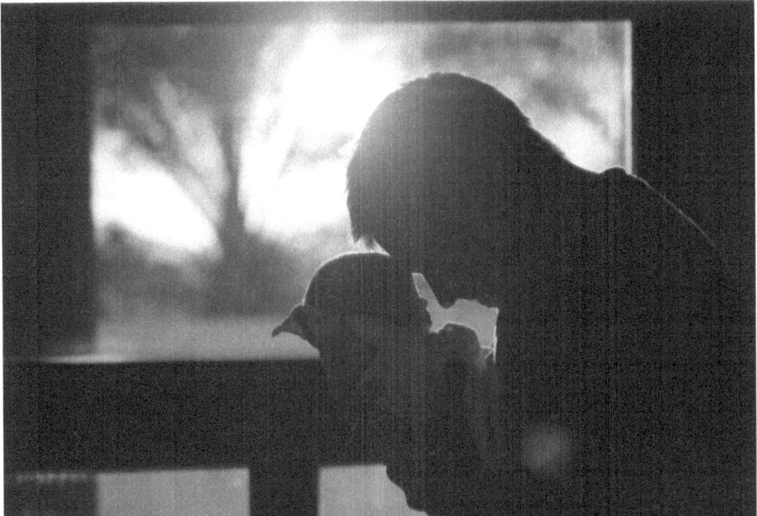

Another easy method that you can use to bond with your child is through communication. This can be through singing your child popular baby songs or just your top ten hits from your favourite playlist. This is how your child will begin to learn more about you and understand their parents. Music is a great tool for your child's cognitive development. Pay attention to how your child responds, as it's not advisable to be blasting music at full volume; this would give you a headache, so imagine what it would do to your newborn. Your approach should always be grounded on being gentle. If you don't consider yourself much of a singer then just talking to your child is more than enough. Watch how your child reacts to your voice and be sure to always make eye contact. Your child needs your attention and eye contact or a simple handhold will do the trick. You will learn what your child enjoys over time by looking at their physical reaction such as a smile, laughter or direct eye contact.

The positioning of your child is important because they require a lot of physical support from you in the early days. It is important to know how to hold your child when generally holding, feeding, sleeping and bathing. When it comes to generally holding your child, it's important to always support your child's head, neck and body. When you first hold your child, the professionals around you are likely to offer a few notes and guide you through it. You can place your child's head in your inner elbow with your arm supporting your baby's body. This is effective depending on the size of your child. If your child is a newborn then two hands are necessary to hold your child one hand under your child's head and one under the child's body. The more you practice holding your child, the more comfortable you will get with it. Always remember how sensitive your newborn is, so it's important to take care when holding them. If you are walking around with your baby, then you can place your child in an upright stance positioning your child's head on your shoulder while you support the head and neck with one arm and the body with the other. It can be nerve-racking at first to allow other people to hold your children out of fear. This is a natural feeling for most new moms as your protective instincts kick in. It is effective to have a few rules in place that apply to everyone who comes into contact with your child. You can require that everyone wash their hands and that for younger children they need to be seated when they hold the baby. This allows your relatives to interact with your child and for other curious children to feel free to play with and get to know your baby. It is important to be protective over your child but allow room for mistakes to happen. The correct positioning for feeding is similar to how you hold your child in the day to day position. When feeding your child it's important to ensure that the position that you are holding them in will not result in choking. This means that your child needs to be held in a more upright position. You can achieve this by placing your child's head on your bicep with your hand on your child's bottom. This will open up your child's airways and prevent choking. Your other hand will be directing the milk to your child. The thought of your child choking is extremely frightening that's why it's important to monitor your child. If your child is unwell, they will express it to you through a cough or by crying.

The next two positions we need to discuss are the right positions for sleeping and bathing. The right position for your child to rest is on their back. This is for a short nap or a full night's rest. It is the most comfortable position for your child in the first few months. It is recommended because it prevents many illnesses from forming. You must be thinking, "But what happens if my child moves around in their sleep and manages to change their position?" You do not have to worry about this because at that stage, they can adjust and maneuver themselves until they are comfortable. You can monitor these movements by looking at your baby monitor. If you would like to monitor your child's sleeping patterns then you can use a portable bassinet or sleeper crib. This allows you to move around with your baby while you do other tasks. It's a great way to calm your anxious feelings in the first few days and continuously spend time with your child. When it comes to bath time, there are a few things your need to remember. The key is that you use a shallow vessel with water, for some people this is a specially made baby bath or it might even be your kitchen sink. The point is to make sure that your child is always being watched and supported. When your child gets older you can add a few extra minutes to bathtime to allow for some monitored play. While water may be an exciting new thing it can also be extremely dangerous (Anon, 2020). This is why many parents decide to teach their children how to swim as early as possible. The water should be lukewarm, you can test this by placing your elbow into the bath. If you aren't sure about the elbow test then you can purchase temperature-sensitive toys. They work by placing them in the water and they change colour when the water is the correct temperature. This prevents you from burning your child's very sensitive skin. The bath shouldn't be too long, so just give your baby a quick gentle wash with a soap that is specifically for new babies. Once you have completed the bath, you can gently lift and place your child in a soft towel. If your child is born in a hospital, then the nurses will show the new parents how to complete bathtime. In some situations, you can just gently wipe your child as opposed to giving a full bath to your baby. You can wipe your child with cotton balls or a soft cloth. Moisturizing your child's skin is very important because it's very soft and sensitive. You should also be aware of what season your child was born in. You will need to take more precautions if your child is born in winter, due to the weather. In the warmer seasons, it's important not to overdress your children because this can cause your child to sweat unnecessarily.

A major part of the first few months just consists of your child feeding, sleeping and needing a diaper change. I think we have all heard the phrase "breast is best" when it comes to feeding your child. The truth is that breastfeeding is extremely difficult for many women. You think that it will be an easy process but the truth is that it can involve many tears and a few unexpected bites from your baby. Your first feed is extremely important if you are not explicitly told by your doctor to not breastfeed. The first feed is important because it is special milk that contains all the nutrients and vitamins that your child requires. Your regular milk will develop at a steady rate depending on the amount of stimulation your nipples receive. You will need to position your breast directly in your child's mouth while they are positioned in an upright stance. This allows your milk to flow easily. If your child is not sucking correctly, then they are likely to get hiccups or begin to cry. If your child seems uncomfortable or they are not being correctly fed then simply repositioning them is often the solution. This can be the position of the child or the angle that you are feeding them at. It is recommended that you breastfeed for a minimum of 3 months. The duration can vary from 3 months up to a few years depending on the mother. Breastfeeding requires the mother to be very vigilant about what she consumes because everything she eats goes to the baby's milk. This means that similarly to during your pregnancy, it is advisable that you don't drink alcohol or smoke any cigarettes. Your diet directly impacts what your child consumes. When you decide to stop breastfeeding, your body will naturally stop producing milk if there isn't any activity for at least a full week. New mommies, remember that your fluids are being drained as your child feeds, so always stay hydrated. There are certain foods that you can eat that help with your lactation. Oatmeal is an easy item that you can incorporate into your diet to help with your milk production. This can be through oatmeal in your breakfast or an easy addition to your daily smoothie. It is a great easy source of iron and fibre. If you find yourself unable to follow your daily routine for breastfeeding either because you weren't home at the time or just because something else just came up, you can try to express your milk using a breast pump. A breast pump is an electric machine that you attach to your breast and it simulates the nipple through a sucking motion that your child would make. This causes your milk to flow into the suction cup that is attached to a baby bottle. You can refrigerate this milk for your child's next feeding. This gives you a bit of freedom and relieves any guilt you might have if you are late for your child's feeding.

A great alternative to breastfeeding your newborn is using a baby bottle and formula. There are specific kinds of milks for each age group, so make sure that you buy the correct one. There are many alternatives depending on what health choices you want to make for your child. You need to take your personal health preferences into consideration when deciding on what option is right for your child. Regardless of what milk you decide to use, understand that breastfeeding does not work for everyone, so it's okay to use formula. You are still a great mother and giving your child all the vitamins and nutrients that they need. Motherhood is not a straight path and many mothers choose to breast-feed and to provide formula simultaneously. Be sure to be well informed about the milk you are using as your child's needs are the most important. Deciding on a baby bottle is as important as deciding on the milk you use. The baby bottle has evolved a lot over the years as they evolve they continue to evolve and become more breast-like. The material used to create the bot-tle also evolved to include more plastic materials that are not toxic. There are a wide range of bottles that are made from glass with some mothers preferring this op-tion, as glass is considered less toxic than plastic. The teet of the bottle should be as close to your breast for the smoothest transition when you stop breastfeeding. This allows your child to strengthen their jaw as they feed.

The materials you use need to be incredibly clean, which is why it's important to sterilize your bottles.

This can be done by purchasing simple sterilizers and following the instructions on its use. The instructions are usually pretty straightforward and this allows you to be cost-effective and correctly use your bottles without putting your child in harm's way. You can alternatively purchase an electric steam sterilizer that is easy and extremely convenient to use. It allows you to complete the many other things that you have to do while your bottles get cleaned. Your bottles should be washed and sterilized every day as it lowers the risk of your child getting sick. You need to consider the temperature of your milk when bottle feeding. A quick way to test the temperature is by splashing a few drops on your inner wrist. If you aren't sure then you can easily buy the thermometer to help you out. This also allows you to be as accurate as possible. You will need to keep track of how much your child eats and the frequency. It will help you form a routine and see what patterns your baby is developing.

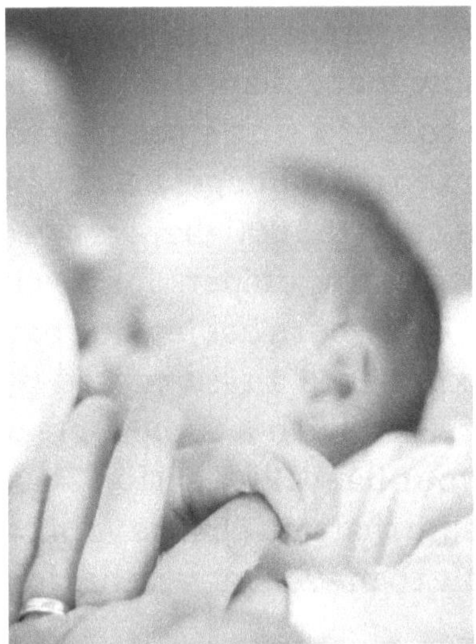

The last major topic that needs to be covered is the dreaded diapers. You will need to get extremely comfortable with changing diapers fairly quickly because your child will be using a lot of them, especially in the first few months. Whether you decide on a disposable diaper or reusable ones they both come with their advantages and disadvantages. It is also important to consider how your child reacts to both options. Whichever side you end up on, just make sure that it suits your lifestyle and it's comfortable for your baby. Disposable diapers are first up on the list. There are many brands to choose from as well as styles. They are advertised as being easy, effective and very convenient because you discard them after one use. Diapers also offer the option of choice with many sizing options depending on the size of your baby.

There are disadvantages to using disposable diapers.

The major disadvantage is the cost of diapers. If you think about how many diapers you will go through in a day and the cost of a single package then the cost is very significant to most budgets. A newborn baby is estimated to use at least 3000 diapers a year if you think about it that's a lot of diapers for a very tiny person (Knisley, 2020). Newborn babies, due to their sensitive skin, might experience a rash caused by the nappies. This can be treated with a topical cream specifically designed for your baby. Prevention is always the best cure so make sure that you change your baby's diaper as soon as possible to prevent any rashes from forming.

The big draw to cloth diapers is that you can reuse them. This helps the moms who are a little more environmentally conscious to do their bit to eliminate waste. They work in conjunction with an internal liner that you put on your baby before wrapping the cloth. The liner is intended to catch the waste and make cleaning up a little easier. You can insert an additional layer with a waterproof top layer in the form of a pull-up bottom in a similar shape to the diaper. You need to be mindful of when you want to change your baby in order to prevent any rashes or discomfort. Cloth diapers are gentler on your baby's skin. The cloth needs to be cleaned after every use or if any leakage has occurred, so make sure that you have at least 20. You'll need to physically remove any feces that have slipped through the liner. This is more of an investment because you will be saving money by reusing these cloths for the early years. You can wash the cloths by hand or in a washing machine depending on what you prefer (The Bump Editors, 2018). When it comes to using either disposable or reusable diapers there are a few items that go hand in hand. You will need baby wipes to help you clean your baby during changes and possibly an additional powder to prevent irritation.

CHAPTER 8: PARENTING HACKS

Parenting hacks are little tips and tricks about things that you might not be aware of already. I highly recommend using these tips throughout your parenting journey in the various stages to help you when you feel a little lost. I will cover a wide range of topics, including things that I've learnt along the way of my own parenting journey.

Firstly, I can't seem to stress this enough, but a routine is a lifesaver. A great way to keep track of your child's behavior is by writing down everything that your child does. This might seem like a lot of unnecessary work or a little extreme, but it helps you better understand what your child is doing and what the current routines are. If you just follow this method for a full week then you can see what your child is doing. It is a simple task that just requires you to write down nap times, feeding times, unexplainable cries and any other behavior that is out of the ordinary. Once you see what the patterns are then you can adjust a few things and try to get your child to sleep throughout the night.

Your baby is very willing to learn especially as they continue to develop. A routine is a great hack to adjust your child's sleeping patterns and eating schedule (Burt Wang, n.d.).

You don't need to wait until your child is ready to attend preschool to start teaching them. Parents have many expectations and plans for their children; many of these include things that they wish they did when they were children. In my case it was ballet lessons, and in yours it might be learning how to play an instrument, speaking a different language, joining a dance class or even just being a more outdoorsy person. These are all great things that we want our children to do, but it's important to not push too many of your desires onto your children. There needs to be room for your child to decide what they want to do and what brings them joy. This is why exposing them to many different things is vital. These might be things that we don't even find remotely interesting but exposure will make your child more confident and aware of the world around them. It is an opportunity to expose them to different cultures and people. Early exposure to things and people that might seem different is very important because it will show your children that every individual is worthy of respect and understanding regardless of the situation. You will raise children who are more socially conscious and understanding of themselves as well as their greater society. These fundamental lessons need to be taught from the very beginning so that your child understands that their actions impact those around them. You want to ensure that the environments that your child is in exposes them to different ideas.

Learning is an ongoing process for not only your child, but for you as well. The lessons should also include helping your child develop language skills before they head off to preschool. This can easily be done through reading to your child and correcting them now and again with the words they use. You can start teaching your child how to count and the alphabet. This will make your child more confident when they start school because the information will not be completely new to them. They will feel more comfortable learning other things because of this. I know you might be thinking, "Well this sounds like a great idea but I'm not a teacher so how am I going to manage to teach my child?" This is a fair fear and all you need to do is lead by example. Your child will copy behaviors that you have and the language that you use in the early stages. You and your partner must be mindful of the language you use and try to speak in complete sentences as much as possible around your child. We all know at least one person who loves to use baby talk and imitate the sounds that babies make. While this is cute it's not very helpful to your child because your child is trying to learn language skills by imitating you. The more words you use, the more stimulus your child receives. This greatly impacts your child's language development. A lesson on consent, personal space and how to freely express your emotions will go a long way in your child's development. When your child is upset, ask them what they are feeling. Is it sadness, happiness, anger or are they just unsure? This helps your child understand reactions as well as equipping them with the words to express how they feel.

Healthy habits start in the very beginning, so a great parenting hack is to start right away and get your child used to following rules and expressing themselves. A healthy habit that you can start is drinking water. Once your child begins to try solid foods and different beverages, the taste of water isn't as exciting as it used to be. This is why it's beneficial to start them early by explaining the benefits of water. You can do this through a song or a demonstration with a plant explaining that plants need water to grow and so do humans. A healthy habit that goes hand in hand with drinking more water is eating healthy meals. If you are a family of meat lovers, try incorporating one vegetarian meal into your diet per week, and giving your children snack options that are either a fruit or a vegetable. A pro tip if your child does not want to eat vegetables: Cut them up into interesting shapes or change their form. You can mash up your vegetables and add them into a meal that your child already loves. The shape and colour can put a child off eating something if you have a picky eater. Invest in a cookie cutter to help make your child's plate look more exciting or try dying the food. I'm not a huge fan of food dying, but if you are out of options then it's worth a try as long as it's a healthy alternative that does not alter the taste. A lovely young mom gave me some advice about getting your children to eat vegetables. If you buy your child a special plate that they love, they will feel great about their food because they get to use their plate every time. This makes your child feel special and gives them something to look forward to. A dessert treat in your household can be a homemade ice cream, a few pieces of fruit or a homemade baked treat that incorporates healthy foods that your child might not always eat.

A great parenting hack is teaching your child about different life processes through a small vegetable patch or flower garden helps your child spend time outdoors and feel a sense of responsibility for another thing. This allows your child to watch something grow and be more patient. They will also understand the importance of plants and where our food comes from. It is important to educate your children about these types of things, because it only further sparks their curiosity about the world they live in. There are many educational programs that you can watch with your child that teaches them about the world around them.

Modern mothers need to be aware of the role that the digital era plays in raising their children. Be mindful of how much screen time your children get and how often you use the screen as a replacement for your attention. Television shows and online programs can be extremely beneficial if used in moderation. Your child needs your care and attention so if you are surprised by unexpected tears, don't run for the television but rather spend time with your child. Long periods of screen time can be unhealthy for developing children. The internet has many dangers, so a great pro tip is to talk to your children about the dangers of the internet and utilize the block feature for certain words to limit their searches. If you have smart devices in your home, you should use the child-friendly options that do not harm your child's development but help facilitate it.

When buying your child clothes, do not fall into the trap of buying absolutely everything just because it looks cute. This type of shopping will likely leave you with financial issues because there will always be another item that is just as tiny and cute. When you shop for clothing, buy the items in various sizes. Your child is growing everyday so if all your items are the smallest available size they will not fit after a few months. The sizes need to vary so that you can get more use out of the items. That doesn't mean that your child needs to drown in clothes that are far too big, but if you buy clothes that are even one size bigger it ends up being a better financial decision. You can either donate the clothes that your child has outgrown or you can keep them in storage if you plan on having more children. It is important to store them in a vacuum-sealed package to properly preserve them. When purchasing toys for your baby, the most important thing you need to consider is the age of your child. In the early days, children put almost everything into their mouths. The toys you buy should not be a choking hazard in any way. This means that toys that have many tiny pieces are not advised in the early days and toys that have many small decorations on them, such as beads that your child can break off, should be avoided. A safe purchase is plush teddy bears, large blocks and large playmats. In the early days it is important to expose your child to different textures and shapes. Here is a great example of toys that are safe for your child at any age:

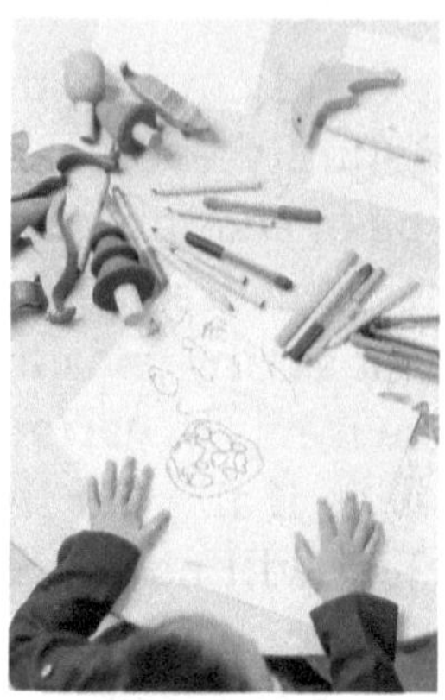

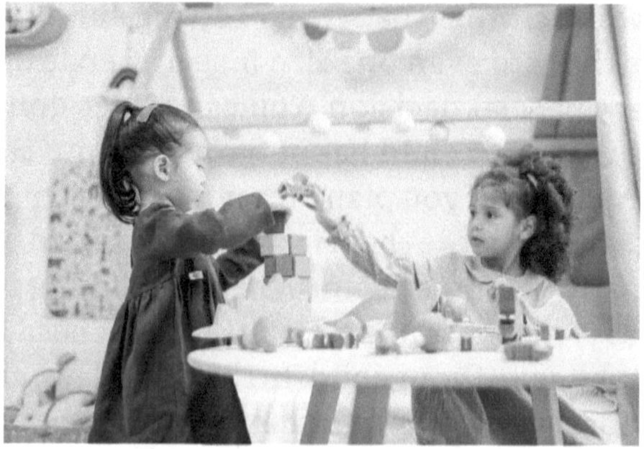

CHAPTER 9: MOTHERHOOD:

Baby Time

Your child's growth and development can be as exciting as it is scary at times. Your child is growing every day from the moment that they are born. These changes might be slight, but after a few weeks it's very normal to only notice the day to day changes. Mommies often say that their children look completely different a few weeks after their birth; this is because for many babies their complexion has changed and they have started to pick up a healthy amount of weight. Everything you do is to try and ensure that your child gets enough love, food and sleep on a daily basis. I will go through what you can expect from each stage of your child's development as well as a few tips on how to enjoy each stage and capture each memory.

In the first few months of your child's life, they require a lot of assistance and support from you as a parent. Your child is incredibly fragile without control over their body movements and functions. It's very normal for parents to not expect many drastic changes from their children at this stage. You should look for the small changes in this stage like a brief smile. Your child will begin to develop control of their arms as they strengthen them by practicing gripping different things. Tummy time is a great activity to strengthen your child's back and muscles. These developments might seem small but they serve as indicators for your child's growth. Your child will develop control over their eyes and you will begin to notice more focused eye contact and different reactions to stimuli. In month four to six, the main changes include your child gaining more strength day in and day out. Your baby will amaze you by sitting up and making more controlled movements. Your home will be filled with infectious laughter and small squeals as your baby begins to, thankfully, do more than cry. Toys that are different shapes and textures help your child greatly during this time as your child uses their hands to understand their surroundings more than ever. Be sure to cut your child's nails because they can harbour a lot of germs and scratch those around them.

In my experience months seven through to ten are the most exciting because they come with your child learning to be more independent. This is the time when your child can confidently move around by crawling. You can help them along by putting their favorite toys in front of them, encouraging them to crawl to them. You need to ensure that your child is crawling on a soft surface. The most noticeable change is your child can start eating soft solid food and even possibly feeding themselves. In the early days, your child might make more of a mess than consume food but they must begin to do things for themselves. You'll notice how excited your child is to hold their spoon, bottle or small snacks. You can start giving them homemade treats or healthy fruit pieces. Teething is a milestone that can start anywhere from six months onward after your child is born. This process can be painful and frustrating for your child, so you might notice more irritable cries and whining. You will notice a change in your child's gums and an unstable need to chew on what seems like everything. You can buy teething tools like teething rings that your child can safely chew on without fear of harming themselves. This also stops your child from sucking on their hands or fingers. You can also purchase teething cookies that are essentially harder biscuits so your child is occupied.

The much anticipated first steps can occur in months ten through to twelve. Parents are always excited about a child's first steps, but you need to understand that especially when it comes to walking, your child might not follow the norm. This does not mean that there is something wrong with your child, because walking varies from baby to baby. In this time, your child can start speaking and interacting with you more by indicating their desires through gestures. Your child might start talking before they start talking or vice versa. Your child will be more playful now and enjoys playing with you more and more. This is because your child is constantly learning from you and seeing your behavior. It's important to speak to your child to help them develop their language abilities and understanding. You can do this by repeating certain words and continuously greeting them by saying hello. This helps your child better understand language and the meaning behind words.

Your child is developing and changing at such a fast pace that it's important to document as much as you can so that you are able to relive these moments. You can start a baby book from conception as you include pictures from your scans. A great way to remember your pregnancy is through a photoshoot to mark the occasion. It's also a great way to remember your time with your baby and build up your confidence. Pregnancy shoots do not need to cost a lot of money to be special, so just think of a theme and maybe look at Pinterest for some inspiration and have it at home. The important thing is that you feel confident and beautiful during the shoot. Here is a great example of a photoshoot concept. You can include notes to your child about your wishes for them as well as how active they were in your belly. Documenting everything lets you see all the changes that are happening and share them later on with your child as they grow older. Your child will appreciate all the pictures, handprints or footprints as they grow older or even when they have their children. This also allows you to remember all that you have been through and the emotions that you were experiencing during this time. A journal is a great way to keep track of your child's growth and development for your child to see in the future. You can write down your child's first words and the date of their first steps. This makes the hard days more worthwhile because you know that there have been positive moments and that there will be more positive moments to come.

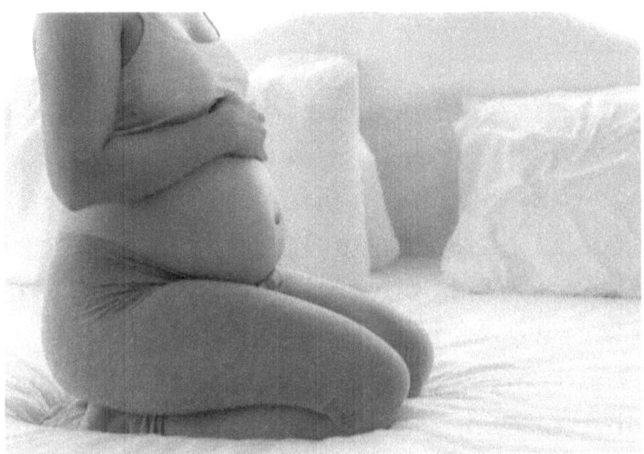

Your child's personality is what makes them uniquely themselves (Smith, n.d.). In the beginning, it might seem like all your child does is cry and occasionally giggle but as time goes on, their personalities become more clear. There are many factors that go into what makes your child who they are and there are a few things that you can do to help the process along. Your child is made up of your genes and that of your partner, this combination is what makes them themselves. Your child's genes influence some key factors in who they are, such as if they are extremely social or not, or if they are innately talkative or not. How you as parents handle your child impacts who they are shaped into. The behaviors that you promote are likely to continue so it is important to strike a balance on the places you push your child while giving them enough room to be themselves. Your child should know that you are dependable and that they can be themselves. It's okay if your child is shy or reserved, you just need to ensure that their nature does not stop them from enjoying themselves. The same can be said if your child is constantly surrounded by people or always need to be the centre of every conversation. It is important to show your child the other side of the coin and that there is room for them to take the backseat at times. You can tell what type of person your child is by seeing how they react to different environments and the people around them. Does your child cling onto you when they enter new environments or are they joyfully running towards other people? It's important to encourage your child to try new things; this is far easier when they are younger because you are their guide. When they continue to grow up, it can become harder to influence their decisions. Your child is their own person so it's okay to allow them to spread their wings. If you promote self-love and a positive self-esteem in your child's younger years then they grow into more self-aware and stronger people.

The way you interact with your child shouldn't be influenced by your child's gender. Gone are the days where blue is only considered for boys and pink is associated with girls. Your child's gender does not play a role in the person that they become. There isn't a right or wrong way to be a boy or girl anymore. This doesn't mean that your little girl will never be a ballerina; it just means that she doesn't have to do it if she doesn't want to. This also means that your little boy might not like sports and that's completely okay. It doesn't make her any less of a girl or any less feminine. It doesn't make him any less of a boy, either, or any less masculine. It is important to acknowledge that there is femininity and masculinity in all of us. You shouldn't feel obligated to put your child in a specific box but rather you should just allow them to be themselves. Your daughter is still your daughter and your son is still your son regardless of their interests. There are studies that believe that girls are innately better at communicating from a younger age as opposed to boys (Smith, n.d.). This same line of thinking believes that boys are less prone to crying and that they can adjust more easily to new environments as opposed to girls. This is due to evolutionary developments that believe that boys needed these differences to be successful hunters. Your child's gender is not directly linked to who they will become or their personalities. Your child will develop fears throughout the years as they begin to understand the world around them. These could include fear of failure, new places or experiences, falling or even noise. These are all normal fears that you should help your child overcome by explaining that it is okay to fear new things. If your child feels supported and that they can trust you then they will be more willing to try new things because they know that you are there to support them. You might have had a plan as to how you would approach parenting your child before they were born, but it's important to consider your child's personality when deciding on how you will interact with them as well as how you will discipline them.

Discipline is a tough topic, as discussed by Karp (2020), for most new parents because they aren't sure about what they need to be doing and when they need to be doing it. I'm sure we all have a horror story or two about getting punished by our parents and we don't want to repeat these behaviors with our children. Gone are the days where spanking is considered the best option or in many cases the only option to discipline your child. Fundamentally, discipline is about teaching your child the difference between right and wrong. If you don't guide your children then they have no way of knowing what the right direction is for them. You should not view discipline as a negative thing, but as a positive way to help your child. There are a few fundamental rules you need to remember when deciding on what your approach should be. You need to consider your child's temperament and personality. If your child is extremely shy then maybe raising your voice is not the best approach as it could force your child to distance themselves. You need to remember that your child is an individual and deserves to be considered and treated with respect. If you want your child to grow into a respectful individual then you need to be their example. The tone you use will impact how your child receives the message and their willingness to receive the message. Your child's age plays a major role in how your child understands discipline and the effectiveness of the method. It's far easier to sit your five year old down and tell them what the issue is or what they did wrong, as opposed to a toddler who might not fully understand what you are trying to convey. Your choice of words will impact the outcome and effectiveness of your method. It is easier to use words that correlate with your child's age such as simple words like "no", "stop" or "danger" for younger children and longer phrases like, "Don't do that", or "That's naughty." You'll find that when your toddler is misbehaving, they are likely to look at you and giggle. Your child usually knows when they are misbehaving so take this opportunity to either not validate this behavior or tell your child to stop. When your child gets older it's helpful to explain to your child why the behavior is bad. Small correction in the early stages can go a long way in how your child grows up. If you set rules for your child then it's important that you stick to them. If you tell your child to not do a certain behavior on Monday, but on Tuesday you allow it, this just confuses your child. Your child will not know what behavior is good or bad if you are inconsistent about how you discipline them (Karp, 2020).

I will provide you with some positive tools that you can use to alter your child's behavior. A great and effective tool that you can use is positive reinforcement. If you reward your child when they clean up after themselves or follow the rules, they are more likely to repeat this behavior. If your child is doing something wrong and you don't reward the behavior, your child will stop the behavior. Your child requires a lot of love and care from you, so if you remove these acts when they are misbehaving it will correct the behavior. You shouldn't be unkind to your child or remove affection for long periods as they can feel rejected by you but you should make it clear when they are behaving badly. A naughty corner or time out is a great option for a toddler, because they can understand what is happening and they will associate the area with what they have done wrong. The corner should be removed from any interaction with others and you should always explain to your child why they are being punished. When you are explaining the issue to your child you should always speak to them at eye level. Your child should know how long they will be in the corner for and you should always be consistent with the duration otherwise it's unfair to the child. Your child should sit in the corner without any toys or communication. Once the timeout is over, tell your child that you are no longer angry with them and physically take them out of the naughty corner. This is an important step because if you leave them in the corner they may feel as though they are still being punished. Rules are important because they keep your child safe and away from any possible dangers around the house. If discipline is difficult for you then remind yourself that you are doing it from a place of love. Rules teach your child about responsibility and how to behave in certain settings.

Household rules are a great way of staying consistent with your discipline methods as your child gets older. You can include your child in these discussions by asking them what they think the rules should include. This will allow rule-making to be a collaborative activity and your child is more likely to follow the rules because they helped create them. The rules should be simple and straightforward to lead to less confusion. A great house rule is: "Above everything we respect all people". This lets your child know that no matter the situation, you treat everyone with respect. This rule will carry into your child's behavior outside of the house. Your reaction should always correspond with your child's behavior. It's important to not overreact when your child does something wrong, but discipline them accordingly. The house rules should also reflect the values that you wish to uphold. These values could be accountability, love, independence, free thinking or respect. There are no right or wrong values; it's important that they work for your family and that they allow your child to be a positive member of society.

CHAPTER 10: MOMMY TIME

Everything flows from you, as the mother, so you need to take care of yourself to be an effective mother and nurture your exciting relationships. Motherhood comes with many pressures, so the pressure must not come from yourself. I chose to make this the last chapter, not because it isn't important, but because I want it to be one of the last things you read. You play a major role in the process as mothers usually feel more attached to their children since they developed inside of their wombs. This is a time to focus on yourself as opposed to your partner or child. I want you to say out loud that you matter and that you are going to put yourself first. It's mommy time.

Scheduling time for yourself can seem extremely difficult in the early days as you are trying to balance your schedule. Your priorities are just trying to make sure that your child is well taken care of. This is not an incorrect approach because your child should come first but I want you to also think of yourself. In the early days, you might be shocked to find that you haven't washed your hair in a week or that you've been wearing the same sweatpants for a full week. Your appearance is the last thing you'll think about or even prioritize. I need you to take some time for your appearance even if it's just a few minutes a day to brush your hair. It might sound silly but a few minutes of just brushing your hair and preparing for the day will impact your outlook of the day. You'll be in a better headspace so you will be able to take better care of your child. You need to prioritize self-care to be successful. There are other small things that you can do to lift your spirits, like making your bath time more enjoyable. You might not have a full hour to soak in the tub but just by playing some light music or lighting a few candles for a 20-minute soak you can feel more energized. A helpful tip is to schedule your baths around your child's naptime. This allows you to take care of yourself without having to wonder about what's happening with your baby. If you keep the baby monitor near you during this time, you can still keep an eye on your child. When your child begins to have a more consistent sleep schedule it will become much easier for you to plan moments for yourself.

Gratitude will play a huge role in this period because you need to remind yourself of how precious every day is. Your child is growing and developing in front of you daily. It can be easy to take this for granted because of increased stress levels of fatigue but you need to remind yourself to be grateful. You can start your morning or finish off your day with a gratitude check by writing down what moment you are grateful for. This can be your child's laughter, a show you enjoyed watching, or even just that you got through the day. A gratitude journal is a great way to look back at what you've been through and the moments that you might have forgotten about. It allows you to recognize how far you and your baby have come. You will experience a different kind of fulfillment from your child that will change your outlook on life. It's important to allow yourself room to grow and develop while still not completely altering your being. If you were a happy person before, then there's no reason why you shouldn't be that now. The aim is not to lose yourself during this transition, but just allowing your personality to develop with you. Gratitude allows you to enjoy the motherhood journey.

A great way to make time for yourself and all the changes that you have experienced is to give yourself a mommy makeover. Your fashion choices will need to be adjusted a little to fit your new body. Your style does not need to change, but you can buy yourself more comfortable alternatives. If you loved constantly wearing jeans that might not be the most comfortable idea straight after giving birth. You can still feel dressed up by switching your jeans for a stylish pair of jeggings. You don't have to say goodbye to your favourite summer dresses, you can just try different styles and cuts to suit your body. You can still be fashionable even as a mother. There has always been this stereotype that mothers have to look a certain way or can't wear certain styles. All these ideas are outdated and there is a consensus that it's perfectly fine for moms to be considered sexy or attractive. Your clothing choices can positively impact how you feel about yourself. Once you have your clothes right then a new hairstyle might be in order. Getting a haircut or colouring your hair is a great way to step out of your comfort zone and introduce yourself as a mom. A haircut that doesn't require a lot of maintenance is a great move for a new mom. We all know that a trip to the hairdresser feels like a form of therapy for many of us, so make the time to go. If you can arrange for your hairdresser to do a home visit that's a great alternative for moms who are not ready to leave the house yet, although a change of scenery is highly recommended. A trip to a day spa or your local manicurist is a fun short trip that can do wonders for your confidence levels. Try treating yourself with a manicure or pedicure once in a while. Just be sure to get a nail shape and length that doesn't impact how you function daily. Claw shaped nails might have been a good idea before you had your baby but now they are probably just going to unintentionally scratch your baby. The main way not to lose yourself in this phase is by finding the time to do the things that you enjoy and finding new hobbies. If you love reading then try reading a chapter a day of a book you love. The point isn't to feel obligated or stressed out about finding windows to pamper yourself, but it's about enjoying this time.

You need to take ownership of your body after pregnancy. The process was affected by your decisions, but you could not completely control the outcome. Your body became a home for a whole other person and once that person moved out, they left a few markers of their presence. It can be hard for you to come to terms with the changes regardless of how excited you are to have a child. You need to be comfortable in your skin, as this can negatively affect your relationship if you do not. This comfort leads to confidence in yourself. Confidence will always be a desirable quality in anyone and more specifically in a first-time mother who trusts in her abilities. Trust me, your partner will be totally attracted to this confidence and assertiveness that you have. A great way to regain your confidence is to spoil yourself with new lingerie. You will be grateful for the new pieces and the confidence that it gives you. Lingerie is another great way to get closer to your partner post-pregnancy. It allows you to be more comfortable with your body and enjoy your new body. Sleep plays a major role in your outlook on life because it impacts how much time to rest your body is getting. Sleep deprivation is very harmful to your mental health and your general physical health. When you are sleep deprived, you are less alert and more likely to intentionally cause harm to yourself or others. Getting enough sleep is an act of self-care because it directly affects your well-being. If you find that you aren't getting enough sleep, then talk to the support system around you about helping out with your child during the day so you can rest for a few hours, or take turns with your partner for nightly feedings.

Self-care includes knowing when to ask those around you for help regardless of what that help is. This could be asking for assistance with your laundry, cooking or just tidying up around your home. You'd be surprised at how quickly your home can feel like a complete mess after a few days of not doing dishes. We live in an age where there is a phone application for anything you can think of. Be sure to use this to your advantage by making your life easier and hiring cleaning services, beauty appointments or grocery deliveries. The idea of hiring someone else to do your household tasks through an application might seem foreign at first but it's a great way to save yourself time. These services are relatively affordable and very easy to book. A great tool you can add to your life is monthly subscription services that can offer you a variety of goods. They range from beauty tools, wine subscription, food deliveries, childrens' products or even clothing. The knowledge that once a month there is something specifically delivered for you is a great way to pamper yourself. I love subscription services because whenever I receive a package it always feels like a gift to myself. This is especially true for subscription services that don't specify what is in their boxes. You will know the general theme but not the specific item. It's a great way to discover new products and services. The wine subscriptions are great for moms who want to host people in their homes. A book club is a great way to socialize with other people who have a similar schedule to you.

Your identity as a mother isn't an overnight switch,

which is why it's important to decide what you want it to be. If it's a conscious decision then you can control your outlook. It helps if you take a moment and take a few moments out of your day to just take stock of how you have adjusted to motherhood; you will be able to see whether or not you are where you want to be. Your situation will not be the same as anyone else's, so it's important to identify your path. Are you a stay at home mom, a working mom or a bit of both. This helps you stay accountable and make time for all the things you want to do. If you want to be a stay at home mom, then you can plan your days around your daily goals and tasks. If you want to stay at home while still making time for your work, then you need to balance out your schedule to suit your needs. It's about finding what works for you and your family. Your identity is who you were before you were a mother and who you want to be after becoming a mother. Your life can seem to centre around your child's needs and wants but you need to not only live for your child but yourself as well. New moms often feel lost because their child's schedule takes precedence above their own. You might feel like all your freedoms have been stripped away but they haven't, you just need to rebalance your mind and change your outlook.

Pressure can come from every corner when it comes to motherhood and pregnancy, but you shouldn't allow it to come from yourself. You need to remember that your baby is an individual who might not reach milestones at the same time that others do. This does not mean that there is anything wrong with your child and you should not allow this to change your attitude towards your child. Your approach will be filled with anxiety or fear, as opposed to joyful and excited. Your child is developing at their own pace so you shouldn't feel pressured by other mothers who love to share every milestone that their children hit. Don't fall into the trap of needing validation from others about your child's developments. This might mean that you need to post less on social media because it negatively affects your outlook or you find yourself comparing your child to others. Focusing on others will simply steal your joy and take moments away from your child. When your child starts walking, you might not be as excited as you should be because instead of being proud of your child, you will be relieved that they finally started walking. Your child's development is a prime example of focusing on your race as opposed to outside influences. You will be at peace once you remove all the pressures that you put on yourself to look a certain way or parent like other people. You are an individual who needs to bring their unique perspectives and thoughts to your parenting style or motherhood journey.

CONCLUSION

Hey Mommy,

I'm so glad that you've taken this journey with me and allowed me to hold your hand throughout this process. We have spoken about everything from mucus plugs, diaper rashes to different discipline methods. There might have been a few things that you had not heard of before, and that's okay. I hope I haven't scared you off but rather that I have given you more information and practical tips and tricks on how to survive your pregnancy and motherhood. Take a moment to think about all the first time moms who are out there and are probably just as scared as you are. This thought often reassured me when I first thought about having children. It is not a decision you should take lightly but the knowledge that many others have done it before you and succeeded is comforting. It lets you know that there is a way to succeed through this journey and helps shape who your children become. Your journey might not be a fairytale, but it is a journey worth taking. Your fears and anxious feelings should now be informed opinions as well as excitement. If anything, by now you should know that children are a huge commitment. It's a lifelong commitment that will surpass any relationship you have because your child is reliant on you. Their beliefs, personality and well-being will be shaped by your actions and the example you set.

Since we have chosen to be open and honest throughout this journey together it shouldn't be a surprise that your commitment to your child starts before conception. You need to make changes to your diet, lifestyle and relationships. All of this is centred around making the necessary changes to accommodate your child. These might seem like drastic sacrifices and changes in the beginning, trust me, I've been there, but knowledge of why you are doing it makes the process worthwhile. It's helpful to start slow, so if you are thinking of trying for a baby then slowly shift your habits to healthier choices. This can look like eating out less frequently, going to the gym once a week to get more active or quitting smoking. If you gradually make these changes they become easier to manage. The most important thing that you need to remember is that the changes are worth it in the end because you want to give your child the best possible start.

The most important lesson that I have learnt is that pregnancy is about getting comfortable with uncertainty. Kids are absolutely little balls of cute chaos and unpredictability. It's something that I realized later on, but I think it's beneficial if you come to terms with it as early on in the process as possible. You might be completely healthy and in optimal condition on paper, but you may have fertility issues. You might try for a child and get pregnant almost immediately but lose the child in the 1st trimester as many women do, you might have planned for a single child but you end up pregnant with twins. These are all deviations from your original regardless of whether they are positive changes or not. The decision to have children is about accepting that you are entering a process that will test you on all levels from your financial stability to your mental strength. You may have considered pregnancy to be an easy process that women should naturally succeed in and for some this is true, but for others the journey is much harder and requires a few adjustments. You should be well-informed about the different routes you can take to reach motherhood. You are still a mother regardless of the method you used to have a child or if the child has your genes. It's important to not compare your journey to anyone else's and especially your child to others.

If you are well informed, then the hurdles that you may stumble upon become easier to navigate past. Planning helps calm your anxious feelings while providing you with a clear plan of action on what you need to consider when wanting to conceive. You will enjoy your pregnancy more if you planned for it as opposed to a surprise pregnancy. Planning also helps you and your partner decide on what your expectations are, as well as opening up a line of honest communication regarding your child. You will appreciate this line because it will allow you both to share your joys and sorrows. This also brings you both closer together in preparation for the pregnancy. This is important because relationship dynamics change after the birth of a child if you both prioritize one another, then it can help both of you stay and feel connected. A solid support system goes a long way in your pregnancy journey regardless of who it is coming from. It can be from a partner, parent, friend or a paid professional. The important thing is that you have someone who you can communicate with.

You want to bring your child into a safe and secure environment where all your focus is on simply raising them. The commitment you make will be continuously rewarded through the different milestones that your child will reach as they grow. Children require active parents who are committed to making them feel loved and appreciated. Your child won't know about the small things that may stress you out on a daily basis. What your child will know is how you were there for them and the different ways you showed them love. Motherhood allows you the opportunity to help shape a person into who they are. This is why your support is necessary because your child can freely express themselves if they know that their mommy is in their corner regardless of if they make a mistake or not. The lessons and values you teach your children through the example and rules that you set will impact the adults that they one day become. This can be a scary thought but as long as you simply try your best every day and show your child the same kindness and respect that you want them to show others, you will be on the right track. If it ever becomes too much for you, then you should consult those around you about what your next steps should be.

Motherhood is no longer a requirement for women to reach at a certain age, so take your time and make the right decision for your life. A good thing to keep in mind is that motherhood is not a death sentence. Your social life, fashion sense, love life or even your hobbies do not need to be completely forgotten. A balanced schedule will allow you to cater to your own needs as well as those of your child. Your life will need to be adjusted but not forgotten. I believe that you will not only survive your pregnancy and motherhood with all its twists and turns but you will find your space and way to thrive. The best way to do that is by making the process your own and parenting in a way that works for you and your new family. It's not an easy process but it is well worth all the ups and downs. You got this!

With love,

A fellow first-time mom

REFERENCES

APHOTOX. (2019). Photo of Baby Girl in Tutu Dress Standing Beside Large Gold Number 1 Balloon. In Pexel.com. Retrieved from [photograph] https://www.pexels.com/photo/photo-of-baby-girl-in-tutu-dress-standing-beside-large-gold-number-1-balloon-2261282/

BabyCentre Medical Advisory Board. (2020). Breathing techniques for labour. Retrieved July 25, 2020, from BabyCentre UK website: https://www.babycentre.co.uk/a544499/breathing-techniques-for-labour

Bath safety: babies and children. (2020). Retrieved July 26, 2020, from Raising Children Network website: https://raisingchildren.net.au/babies/safety/bath-water-safety/bath-safety

Besich, B., & Hochwald, L. (2020). Water Birth: Pros, Cons, and What You Need to Know. Retrieved from Parents website: https://www.parents.com/pregnancy/giving-birth/vaginal/what-is-water-birth/

Braaksma, H. (n.d.). 15 Baby Nursery Must-Haves: Your Essential Checklist. Retrieved from Parenting website: https://www.parenting.com/decor/baby-nursery-essentials-checklist/

Broadwell, L. (2002, September 5). 8 Tips for Choosing Child Care. Retrieved from Parents website: https://www.parents.com/baby/childcare/basics/8-tips-for-choosing-child-care/

Burt Wang, J. (n.d.). Why Is Routine Important for Babies? Making and Keeping Routines, Plus What to Do When Routines Are Interrupted. Retrieved July 26, 2020, from Parents website: https://www.parents.com/baby/care/newborn/why-is-routine-important-for-babies/

Centers for disease control and prevention. (2019). Preventing Pregnancy-Related Deaths | CDC. Retrieved from www.cdc.gov website: https://www.cdc.gov/reproductivehealth/maternal-mortality/preventing-pregnancy-related-deaths.html

Corrigan, C. P., Kwasky, A. N., & Groh, C. J. (2015). Social Support, Postpartum Depression, and Professional Assistance: A Survey of Mothers in the Midwestern United States. The Journal of Perinatal Education, 24(1), 48–60. https://doi.org/10.1891/1058-1243.24.1.48

Cottonbro. (2020). Child Holding Brown and Green Wooden Animal Toys. In Pexel. Retrieved from [photograph] https://www.pexels.com/photo/child-holding-brown-and-green-wooden-animal-toys-3661264/

de Bellefonds, C. (2018). Working out When You're Trying to Get Pregnant. Retrieved from What to Expect website: https://www.whattoexpect.com/getting-pregnant/health-and-wellness/safeguard-your-health/exercise-before-pregnancy.aspx

DeNoon, D. J. (2010). Smokers' Sperm Less Fertile. Retrieved from WebMD website: https://www.webmd.com/smoking-cessation/news/20100910/smokers-sperm-less-fertile#1

Fertility, Y. (2012). Exercise may help with conception, study finds | Your Fertility. Retrieved July 16, 2020, from www.yourfertility.org.au website: https://www.yourfertility.org.au/latest-news/exercise-may-help-conception-study-finds

freestocks. (2016). Basinet and teddy bear mobile. In Unsplash. Retrieved from https://unsplash.com/photos/sVwzvlpeEAU/info

freestocks. (2017). baby birthday. In Unsplash. Retrieved from [photograph] https://unsplash.com/photos/qlS6vMR2PpU

Gebauer-Steinick, K. (2020). 11 Bonding Benefits of Skin-to-Skin Kangaroo Care. Retrieved July 17, 2020, from Unitypoint.org website: https://www.unitypoint.org/livewell/article.aspx?id=220158f5-1880-40da-9dcb-8f13f30aa983

Green, A. (2018). How prenatal counselling can help you through pregnancy. Retrieved July 12, 2020, from Today's Parent website: https://

www.todaysparent.com/pregnancy/pregnancy-health/how-prenatal-counselling-can-help-you-through-pregnancy/

Hartshorn, J., & Tomlin, C. (n.d.). 7 Tips for Creating a Newborn Photoshoot at Home. Retrieved July 26, 2020, from Parents website: https://www.parents.com/fun/entertainment/gadgets/tips-to-improve-baby-pictures/

Karp, H. (n.d.). How to Discipline a Child. Retrieved July 26, 2020, from Happiest Baby website: https://www.happiestbaby.com/blogs/toddler/when-does-discipline-begin

Kashtan, P. (2019). Hospital Bag Checklist: What to Pack in Hospital Bag. Retrieved July 25, 2020, from www.thebump.com website: https://www.thebump.com/a/checklist-packing-a-hospital-bag

Knisley, K. (2020). How Many Diapers Do I Need? A Guide to Stocking Up. Retrieved from Healthline website: https://www.healthline.com/health/baby/how-many-newborn-diapers-do-i-need

Magher, M. (2017). Can You Leave the Hospital Without Naming Your Baby? Hello Motherhood. Retrieved from https://www.hellomotherhood.com/can-leave-hospital-naming-baby-18542.html

Marcin, A. (2018). Hair Loss in Pregnancy: Treatment, Causes, and What to Expect. Retrieved July 26, 2020, from Healthline website: https://www.

healthline.com/health/hair-loss-in-pregnancy

Masters, M. (2018). The Pre Pregnancy Diet. Retrieved July 11, 2020, from What to Expect website: https://www.whattoexpect.com/getting-pregnant/health-and-wellness/foods-to-enjoy/prepregnancy-diet.aspx

Mayo clinic Staff. (2019). In vitro fertilization (IVF) - Mayo Clinic. Retrieved from Mayoclinic.org website: https://www.mayoclinic.org/tests-procedures/in-vitro-fertilization/about/pac-20384716

McWhinney, J. (2020). Top 6 Marriage-Killing Money Issues. Retrieved July 13, 2020, from Investopedia website: https://www.investopedia.com/articles/pf/09/marriage-killing-money-issues.asp

Merriam-Webster. (2020). Fertility. In Merriam-Webster. Retrieved from https://www.merriam-webster.com/dictionary/fertility

Nappy. (2020). Man in Gray Shirt Holding Baby in White Onesie. In Pexels. Retrieved from [photograph] https://www.pexels.com/photo/man-in-gray-shirt-holding-baby-in-white-onesie-3536630/

Planned Parenthood. (2019). Planned Parenthood. Retrieved from Plannedparenthood.org website: https://www.plannedparenthood.org/learn/pregnancy/miscarriage

Piceli, G. (2019). Pregnant Woman Wearing White Skirt Holding Her Tummy. In *Pexel*. Retrieved from https://www.pexels.com/photo/pregnant-woman-wearing-white-skirt-holding-her-tummy-2100337/

Rebecca Buffum Taylor. (2011). Using a Surrogate Mother: What You Need to Know. Retrieved from WebMD website: https://www.webmd.com/infertility-and-reproduction/guide/using-surrogate-mother#2

Rivard, M. (2017). Why Adoption is Important for Everyone. Retrieved July 12, 2020, from adoption.com website: https://adoption.com/why-adoption-is-important-for-everyone

Salgado, I. (2016). How to plan financially for a baby. Retrieved July 25, 2020, from Parent website: https://www.parent24.com/Family/Finance_Legal/How-to-plan-financially-for-a-baby-20150826

Shevtsova, S. (2018). Photo of green salad. In Pexels.com. Retrieved from [photograph] https://www.pexels.com/photo/photo-of-green-salad-4117679/

Sick kids Staff. (2016). AboutKidsHealth. Retrieved July 16, 2020, from www.aboutkidshealth.ca

website: https://www.aboutkidshealth.ca/Article?contentid=1989&language=English

Sidekix Media, S. M. (2020). Nursery. In Unsplash. Retrieved from [photograph] https://unsplash.com/photos/AV2tGobH2FM

Sikkema, k. (2019). Black Android smartphone. In Unsplash. Retrieved from [photograph] https://unsplash.com/photos/SBxdMoOY9zM

Smith, E. (n.d.). Understanding Your Baby's Personality. Retrieved July 26, 2020, from Parents website: https://www.parents.com/baby/development/social/understanding-babys-personality/?slide=slide_5a7766bc-9161-4560-b52b-f5f04d7817ed#slide_5a7766bc-9161-4560-b52b-f5f04d7817ed

Stanway, P., & Lousada, S. (2000). MOTHERCARE new guide to pregnancy and babycare: from conception to age five (p. 14). London, Lon.: Conran Octopus.

Tankilevitch, P. (2020). Crop mother playing with baby. In Unsplash. Retrieved from [photograph] https://unsplash.com/photos/if29-uf4N_Q

Tankilevitch, P. (2020). Cute toddler playing with wooden rattle. In Pexel. Retrieved from [photograph] https://www.pexels.com/photo/cute-toddler-playing-with-wooden-rattle-3875217/

The Bump Editors. (2018). Diaper Decisions: Cloth Diapers vs. Disposable. Retrieved

July 20, 2020, from Thebump.com website: https://www.thebump.com/a/cloth-diapers-vs-disposable

University of Utah staff. (2009). Hormone Therapy and Fertility. Retrieved from healthcare.utah.edu website: https://healthcare.utah.edu/healthfeed/postings/2019/04/estrogen.php

Vercelletto, C. (2018). Baby Classes' Benefits. Retrieved from Nymetroparents.com website: https://www.nymetroparents.com/article/benefits-of-group-classes-for-babies

Webster, M. (2020). Pregnant. In Merriam-Webster. Retrieved from https://www.merriam-webster.com/dictionary/pregnant#h1

Westaway, B. (2016). The BMI Explained: How Useful Is It Really? Huffington Post. Retrieved from https://www.huffingtonpost.com.au/2016/02/05/bmi-explainer-obesity_n_9165170.ht